D0017466

What Is **He** Thinking??

ALSO BY REBECCA ST. JAMES

Sister Freaks
Pure
Loved

Available from FaithWords wherever books are sold.

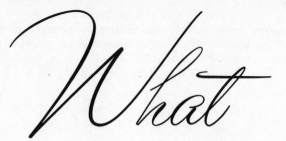

Is **He**

Thinking??

WHAT GUYS WANT US TO KNOW ABOUT DATING, LOVE, AND MARRIAGE

Rebecca
St. James

NEW YORK   NASHVILLE   BOSTON

Copyright © 2011 by Rebecca St. James
All rights reserved. Except as permitted under the U.S. Copyright Act of 1976,
no part of this publication may be reproduced, distributed, or transmitted in
any form or by any means, or stored in a database or retrieval system,
without the prior written permission of the publisher.

All Scripture quotations, unless otherwise indicated, are taken from the HOLY BIBLE,
NEW INTERNATIONAL VERSION®. NIV®. Copyright © 1973, 1978, 1984 by Biblica, Inc™.
Used by permission of Zondervan. All rights reserved.

Scripture quotations marked NASB are taken from the *New American Standard Bible*.
Copyright © 1960, 1962, 1963, 1968, 1971, 1972, 1973, 1975, 1977, 1995 by The Lockman
Foundation. Used by permission. (www.Lockman.org). All rights reserved.

Scripture quotations marked NLT are taken from the Holy Bible, *New Living
Translation*, second edition. Copyright © 1996, 2004. Used by permission of Tyndale
House Publishers, Inc., Wheaton, Illinois 60189. All rights reserved.

Scripture quotations marked *The Message* are taken from *The Message*.
Copyright © 1993, 1994, 1995, 1996, 2000, 2001, 2002 by NavPress Publishing Group.
Used by permission. All rights reserved.

FaithWords
Hachette Book Group
237 Park Avenue
New York, NY 10017

www.faithwords.com

Printed in the United States of America

First Edition: September 2011
10 9 8 7 6 5 4 3 2

FaithWords is a division of Hachette Book Group, Inc.
The FaithWords name and logo are trademarks of Hachette Book Group, Inc.

The publisher is not responsible for websites (or their content) that are not
owned by the publisher.

Library of Congress Cataloging-in-Publication Data
St. James, Rebecca.
    What is he thinking?? : what guys want us to know about dating, love,
and marriage / Rebecca St. James.—1st ed.
        p. cm.
    ISBN 978-0-446-57267-5
    1. Man-woman relationships—Religious aspects—Christianity. 2. Single
people—Conduct of life. 3. Dating (Social customs)—Religious aspects—
Christianity. 4. Marriage—Religious aspects—Christianity. I. Title.
II. Title: What guys want us to know about dating, love, and marriage.
    BT705.8.S7 2011
    241'.6765—dc22
                                                                    2011003699

I dedicate this book to the guys I've dated. Thanks for being used by God in my life. And thanks for motivating long conversations with my gal friends as we try to figure you guys out. You have inspired this book!

God, I dedicate these pages to You. May You use this book to encourage . . . as I have been encouraged.

❧ Contents ❧

❧ Acknowledgments ❧

First of all, a massive thank-you to a guy who knows that without him this book would not be what it is—and perhaps not be at all. You know who you are and I am exceedingly grateful for you.

To Julian, Jon, Shawn, Stein, Robbie, Nick, Garret, Nathan, Willie, Jeff, Brendon, Cale, Andrew, Justin, Bradley, and Brandon. You guys are a huge blessing and encouragement. Thanks for being open with me about this minefield of a topic and for being used to bless others through this book.

Thanks to Dad, Daniel, Ben, Joel, Luke, and Josh for being examples of godly men to me and for holding the standard high!

Thanks to all the "married ones" who let me use your words and advice in this book...you are living legends.

Thanks to my BFF Karleen, to Vicky, Evie, Joel, Lila, Ash, and Jen; and to my mum, Helen, and sis, Libby, for letting me laugh and cry on your shoulders about boys.

To Andrea at Alive Communications for your incredible support and understanding when it came to this book, from that first lunch about it in San Diego!

Thank you to the wonderful team at FaithWords, especially Rolf! Thanks for listening to my idea during the hubbub at ICRS and for supporting me so beautifully throughout the years.

And more than anyone I want to thank my amazing husband (of just a few months!) Jacob. What a privilege it is to belong in marriage to you! I am over the moon that I get to be by your side as we travel this adventure called life...together! Words cannot describe the joy it is to be your wife, your best friend, and your helpmate. Thank you for your cherishing love—you are an amazing gift of God.

Jesus, thank You for being the author of love. Thank You for giving us language with which to connect and share our hearts. Guide us all as we pursue relationships that honor You. We are Yours.

✦ Introduction ✦

I grew up in a home with five younger brothers, so I may have a head start on this topic of guys and what they're thinking. Then again, when it comes to understanding guys in the romantic arena, sometimes I feel like I have absolutely no clue. Can you relate? If you're a Christ follower and have dated any guys, has it ever seemed as if you were navigating a minefield? That's how dating for Christians can sometimes feel. It can be tough out there, and lots of questions are racing through our minds...about our identity, about guys, about what God thinks of all this. *How much should we pursue in a relationship, and how much should we wait to be pursued? What about Internet dating? Is it still possible in our culture today to maintain physical and mental purity? Are there any good guys left? If so, why haven't they stepped up?* When I started researching for this book, I was very excited about its premise. I would seek to find out what guys really think about dating, love, and marriage simply by asking them...a few of my friends, at least.

THE PROCESS

Over a period of four months I conducted interviews with sixteen single guys, ages eighteen to thirty-five. I'm extremely grateful to my friends for allowing themselves to be put on the hot seat. They all did an awesome job. I asked them to be open and honest, and they were. They said some things that we need to hear, girls.

Then I talked with eleven married men to get their take on

some of the same questions I asked the single guys. And especially concerning all things that deal with married bliss. *Is it still possible to find a mate today and live happily ever after?* I desperately wanted to know what they think about that question and more from their perspective—on the other side of the fence. I trust you'll enjoy what they have to say as well.

CHOOSING THE GUYS

I started with a list of about thirty single guys I know and respect, who hope to find a life partner someday. I was curious what insight they would give concerning what this generation of men thinks about dating and marriage, and how they relate to the single women in their lives who are waiting for "Mr. Right." I was hoping for a combination of high-profile men and "guys next door," so we could hear from a few different perspectives. I also wanted to include some words of wisdom from older men I admire and respect—mentors who have been successfully married for years—people like my dad, a pastor I know, a former bandmate of mine, and "taken" men who are seeking after God. I wanted to give them the floor to say what they'd really like women to know.

Due to time and accessibility of all involved, I quickly learned that I had to limit the amount of interviews I would conduct. The questions I asked and the responses they gave have shaped the book that you hold in your hands. I prayed that God would direct me to the right guys to interview, and I believe that He did.

I'm very pleased with the results. I hope that you will see these men (and those in your life who are seeking God) as brothers in Christ. I pray that God will take the words they have shared and help you apply the truths to your life in a way in which He sees fit—according to His perfect plan.

CHOOSING THE QUESTIONS

I was very curious about what guys think about first dates, what is attractive to them, big-time turnoffs, setting physical boundaries, connecting with a girl on an emotional and spiritual level, and so on. Lots of questions swirled around in my head. I called, texted, and e-mailed some of my closest girlfriends to get their opinions on what I should ask. My list of potential questions grew into the hundreds. It was a challenge selecting just the right questions to ask individual guys. Again, I prayed to God, asking for His direction on the matter. I wanted to ask some fun, lighthearted questions, some deep and challenging questions, some easy, some hard. Some questions I asked of almost all of the guys. Some I asked only of a few.

THE RESULTS

Along the way I'll share some surprises, things I learned about myself, preconceived ideas that were confirmed... or denied. And I'll share some stories. A lot of their stories. And stories from my own dating life. My hope and prayer is that this will be very helpful to you as my sister in Christ.

I've lost track of the amount of times I've been the interviewee over the years—for magazines, on radio and TV, and on stage during concerts. It was fun for me to turn the tables and be the *interviewer* this time around, and I had an absolute blast doing it! I hope you enjoy coming along with me on this journey. Ready to dive in? Let's go! Let's see what guys really think.

Rebecca St. James

What
Is He
Thinking??

1

First Impressions

WHAT ARE GUYS *REALLY* LOOKING FOR?

"Your beauty should not come from outward adornment, such as braided hair and the wearing of gold jewelry and fine clothes. Instead, it should be that of your inner self, the unfading beauty of a gentle and quiet spirit, which is of great worth in God's sight."

—1 Peter 3:3–4, NIV

Dating is a bit like diving in the deep end. Sometimes you've just gotta throw yourself in.

When I was five years old until I was around seven, I took swimming lessons. It always occurred when we were on school vacation at Christmastime, which is when we had hot weather in Australia. My parents, aunts, and uncles figured that was a good time for all of us cousins to learn to swim. The problem for us was that the pool was cold. On top of that, it was an ocean pool, which meant that crabs (and maybe sharks!) could have jumped in there during the night. Needless to say, my cousins, siblings, and I were not happy about these swimming lessons. Our teacher Ronnie would have us dive off the diving board into the deep pool.

I'm convinced the diving board was six feet from the surface of the water. Okay, maybe it was only four, but it felt like ten!

At the end of the day, the prizes we received after our cold and scary swimming lessons made the pain all worth it. Ronnie sang songs to us, swung us round and round on the surface of the water, and then we got lollies (candy). Ah. Worth it.

Dating often feels so threatening, doesn't it? It's like being put to the test, over and over again. Braving the potentially cold, possibly shark-ridden waters of relationships can be ultra scary. But let's face it . . . it's worth it. The joys of dating, the lessons learned, and the potential life mate that will come of it are the lollies, music, and spinning ride of dating. Fear must be put aside. My mentor reminded me not too long ago of something the apostle John said: "There is no fear in love. But perfect love drives out fear" (1 John 4:18). We cannot let fear reign in our dating decisions.

FUN TIMES!

Like many other things in life, the dating experience is full of ups and downs, lessons to be learned, and things to discover about yourself, God, and others. I've learned plenty and have had some interesting stories to tell along the way. For instance, I was once asked by my date to jump into a smelly, polluted lake with him at night. I said no. My adventurous side kind of wanted to, but I'm quite sure if you had smelled that lake you would have said no too! Another time, while I was living in Nashville, Tennessee, a guy took me to Pancake Pantry (a legendary Nashville tradition) to pick up some pancakes and eat them in a nearby park. I absolutely loved it! I asked some of my guy friends about their dating stories—both fun and embarrassing moments. Here's some of what they had to say.

Julian Bailey was the guinea pig—my first interview for this book. He's thirty-three, an actor, musician, and lover of Jesus!

We've been friends for nearly three years. We both have a passion for being involved in faith-based films in Hollywood. We got to act together in the movie *Sarah's Choice,* where we had to pretend like we were dating. We even had to practice kissing! I asked him about fun dates. "One time I met a girl at a party and there were some leftovers from the food that was served there. After everybody left, she wanted to go out and give the food away to homeless people. I thought that was really cool and showed me something of her heart. I think a fun time out would be any situation in which we really connect and have fun, do crazy stuff on a whim, whatever is going on in the moment."

My friend Nathan Postlethwait is also thirty-three years old and lives in California. He's done a number of things in his life so far, from pharmaceutical sales to a Realtor business to working at a design firm. Nathan was my next-door neighbor in Franklin, Tennessee, for a while and loves great conversations, painting, and good books. Here are some of his ideas for fun dates:

- Go for a run on the beach and grab breakfast near the water.
- Go to an art museum together.
- Go to a park and pretend that you are little kids, playing on the swings and monkey bars.

I toured with my friend Jeff Bowders for two and half years. He's a drummer who lives in Los Angeles, travels the world playing, and teaches at a music school called Musicians Institute. Once, the band and I about died laughing when Jeff pretended to flirt with some nuns in a European airport shuttle! Good thing they didn't speak English. Here's what Jeff had to say: "I love going on hikes that take you deep into no-man's-land, crossing creeks, etc. I'm a fan of random road trips. I'd rather go husk corn in Nebraska than go to the Grand Canyon." Some other ideas he shared include:

SOME OF REBECCA'S RANDOM DATING STORIES

- I once sketched a drawing of a lion for the guy I was seeing at the time. It was in the style of *The Lion King.* I do not draw, but this was a very special occasion. He cried when I gave it to him.
- A guy I dated very briefly once wrote a prophetic poem for me. He was a singer/writer for a living, so it was beautifully written and powerful.
- I took a guy to a lookout at night just to see the view. Seriously. Well, maybe I thought it would be a romantic moment. The view was interrupted by power lines, it turned out to be very cold up there…and it was unromantic instead.
- I've gone bike riding and have sat on the handlebars while the guy pedaled the bike.
- I like rollerblading with my date.
- I've prayed with a date while on a mountaintop.

"Get a haircut together. Walk through tide pools at Laguna Beach. And going kayaking is awesome!"

I met Andrew Naffin while I was on a study break in 2004 at L'Abri in the beautiful Swiss Alps. Andrew is twenty-eight years old, got a business degree at Washington State in Vancouver, and attended seminary at Gordon-Conwell. He loves reading, fishing in Alaska, and being outdoors.

Fun dates according to Andrew? "Going to bookstores, browsing around for one book to buy each, then going to a coffee shop afterward, relaxing and reading our books. I also like hiking, backpacking, and having a picnic—and you can read books to each other there. I've also gone kayaking with a date. It's fun being outside and doing some active things together. It's fun to see how people respond to physical challenges that push you— like rock climbing." He continues, "I've also gone on a ferry ride with a date. Getting dressed up and going out to a fancy dinner also has its place. It can be very fun and magical. Another idea: pick a unique place in town that you haven't been to before and go to some quaint shops. Both of you look for something small but meaningful to give to the other person at the end of the date."

Here are a few crazy things I told Andrew I've done before on dates. I went to a card shop with a guy and we found cards that made us think of each other. We'd each "give" by showing them to the other person, even though we didn't actually buy and give them. Fun...and cheap! I've also had a "question of the day" that both people respond to, to intentionally explore parts of the other person's heart. Not something I'd recommend for a first date, however!

My friend Cale Wright is eighteen years old, just graduated from high school, and attending Biola University. He likes snowboarding and plays bass, piano, guitar, and ukulele. He lives outside San Diego. Here are some fun dates he'd like to try: "At night San Diego is really awesome, so I'd take my date to a nice Italian restaurant, then walk the city. Tandem bike riding is pretty cool. And I'd go to art museums."

FIVE DATE QUESTIONS YOU HAVE TO ASK (ACCORDING TO EHARMONY.COM)

Caution: Don't slap the list on the table and start jotting down notes. It's a date, not *Jeopardy!*

1. What's your favorite book/movie/TV show this year?
2. Where would you live if you could live anywhere?
3. What would be your ideal job?
4. Who's your best friend?
5. Do you have any hobbies?[1]

Garret Rutherford, from Atlanta, Georgia, is thirty-four years old and a marketing consultant for Chick-fil-A, Coke, and other major corporations. Garret is a dear family friend, has a terrific sense of humor, and loves to say "my pleasure" without anyone thanking him for anything. I loved what he said: "If there was laughing involved on the first date, it was a good date for me."

THE MARRIED GUYS SPEAK

I asked several of the married guys this question, "How did you keep your dating life fun?" Here's what a few of them said. My friend Steve Conrad, who used to play bass in my band, responded, "I tried to always think of creative dates. We generally didn't do the 'dinner and a movie' option (although there's nothing wrong with that every once in a while). Emily loved that each date was an adventure—doing new and unexpected things (like going to the rodeo or going apple picking), and these dates made for great memories that we still treasure today."

I have a tremendous amount of respect for Ted Baehr, who is president of Movieguide. I've sung at and hosted parts of their awards ceremony in L.A. a few times. Ted reminisces, "Our dating life was full of travel, acting classes at the Lee Strasberg Institute, interesting meetings with renowned, very famous individuals, and wonderful opportunities to do God's work."

My cousin Matt Smallbone (who's married) had some great things to say about first impressions. Here are three quick take-aways he wanted me to share with you:

1. A guy can like you in one second. It just happens. Men are wired that way. Take it as a compliment.
2. Chill out. Be a fun date. Everyone enjoys hanging out with fun people. A confident girl who can laugh at stuff (and

herself) is refreshing. No one wants to be bored. The happiest marriages I know are characterized by lots of laughter.

3. Be flexible with paying for dinner. I always appreciated it when a girl offered to pay half. It allowed me to say, "No thanks, I've got it." My future wife had a good job before I did, so she often covered the meal. It was cool.

WHAT THEY'RE LOOKING FOR

So what exactly are guys looking for in women that makes us worth pursuing? Obviously, a physical attraction has to be there. But what else are they looking for? Here's how I asked Julian.

REBECCA: Think about different girls you've been drawn to over the years. Apart from the physical attraction, what made them stand out? For me, it might be a combination of confidence or gentleness or the love of God that shines through his eyes. There's another level of connection, because there is a spiritual and an emotional element. What is that for you?

JULIAN: Apart from physical attraction, one is relatability, feeling like there is a communication connection, grounded or rooted in some kind of soul connection. Maybe there is a gifting or calling or a similar heart. Another thing is a sense of humor for me; someone that gets my jokes. Personally, I like girls who don't talk too much. Some people have the need to fill in all the blanks. I like it when there's give and take. On the other hand, some girls don't talk about anything.

REBECCA: I went to an improv class for a while. It was so fun! The major principle of improv is "yes... and..." You are listening to and accepting what the other person is saying, and then adding to it. That's a good relational goal—to listen and then add to what the other person is saying.

JULIAN: On a spiritual level, something that draws me to a girl is that she is engaged in worship to God and doesn't seem bothered by others around her. She has an obvious, simple faith, and isn't trying to impress anyone.

REBECCA: On a scale of 1 to 10, how much is based on pure physical attractiveness, the outward appearance? (At an initial meeting, for me it's maybe a 7.)

JULIAN: It's very important, probably a 10. It is one of the top things...but I think the inner beauty and character can actually affect how a girl looks on the outside.

We had just finished doing a show and I was talking backstage with Jon Patton, nineteen, a really godly young man who recently got engaged. I asked him, "What do you find beautiful in a woman?"

He said, "Besides the physical beauty, I look for a desire to please God and a heart that loves people. Bigheadedness is such a turnoff. It's not about you, it's about other people—and that's beautiful to me! I admire someone who is caring, graceful, and respectful."

Brendon Shirley and I went to the same church for several years and served on the worship team together a few times. He is twenty-six, a God-honoring man and a gifted musician. I was lucky to have him out on the road with me as my keyboard player. I asked, "What are the three most attractive qualities in a woman?"

Definitely humility, a sweet servant spirit, but with a little bit of spunk and sassiness (but not too much!). Girls who are willing to serve behind the scenes and not get much recognition show their character. And number three...something else that makes a girl really stand out is how she treats other girls while she is face to face with them. Is what she says about them behind their backs consistent with how she treats them face to face? And how does a girl handle how people have hurt her? Does she handle it with grace? She doesn't have to be superwoman, but if she talks trash about people, then that says a lot about her character (sort of like the movie *Mean Girls*).

Shawn Thomas, twenty-five, is an actor friend of mine that I know through a philosophy group I attend. Shawn is a deep thinker, very expressive, and kind. And he gives the most amazing hugs! He lives in L.A. and wasn't raised as a Christian, but became one just three years ago through an arts community. I asked him, "After becoming a Christian, do you feel like what you're looking for now is different than what you were looking for in a girl before?"

Shawn immediately remarked, "Without a doubt. Before I couldn't quite put my finger on what would attract me to a girl. Obviously, there had to be a natural physical attraction. I always was a big fan of a girl who had her own story and had a lot of life experience—someone who was very comfortable in her own skin. And a girl who had a very free spirit, someone who could roll with life and wasn't very high maintenance. Sense of humor was also very important...the ability to laugh at life and not take yourself too seriously. These things all carried over to now." He paused. "But I also found myself being drawn to women who tended to have problems. I wanted someone who understood some tough stuff, because I had had some difficult stuff as well."

When I asked Shawn about the top three qualities (besides physical attractiveness) he's looking for in a woman, he answered,

It's easy to be beautiful on the outside, based on God-given attributes. But to be a great human being takes a lot of work. Some of the words that come to mind are a true nurturing grace—to stay tender in your femininity. Sexuality is so powerful, but within the

Christian context it can be seen as a shameful thing. I'm looking for "godly sexuality," which is a very tricky thing.... You are His bride, and He pursues you passionately. You don't just give physical intimacy away to anyone, it has to be within the context of what God desires for you in marriage. Not having sex before marriage is not "denying natural feelings"—it is actually growing it into what it should become in marriage. It is a powerful gift that you are going to share with the man you marry.

"Oh," Shawn said, "and the last thing is a sense of humor."

Robbie Baehr, twenty-five, is a guy friend I met through my roommate. We both attended a young adults event at a church in L.A. for a while. He is involved in full-time ministry with an organization that supports clean, quality movies in Hollywood. He is looking for someone whose "faith is the most important. She should also be intellectually interesting, someone who is passionate about things, someone who can communicate with others well, someone who comes from a good family, someone who is pretty." Robbie is in sales and loves this quote that could possibly be applied to dating as well: "In sales you either make an excuse or you find a way."

Like Shawn, I also know Stein Willanger (who is thirty-one) through my philosophy group. He has modeled for a few years and started a clothing label. He did some acting, but now he is a screenwriter. Here's his response when I asked about the top characteristics he's looking for in a woman: "Somebody who is a truth seeker, is confident without betraying humility, someone who knows how to laugh and goof around (and doesn't take herself too seriously), someone who is truly introspective (self-analytical) and doesn't just think she is, an engaging conversationalist for the love of God, physically attractive and likes to work out."

MY TOP FIVE TRAITS IN A GUY
(IN NO PARTICULAR ORDER)

1. Physical attraction.
2. Sense of humor.
3. Kindness.
4. A good communicator.
5. A lover of Jesus.

Side note: My brothers came up with the phrase "holy honey" to describe what they're looking for!

I first met Nick Vujucic in 1997 or 1998. He is from my homeland of Australia, and he has a very powerful story. For reasons nobody knows, Nick was born with no arms or legs. He wanted to believe that God was a loving God, but he didn't know why this happened to him. He asked God for a "plan B" as a child, but God never gave him more than a "plan A." He experienced a very deep depression between ages eight and twelve, and tried to commit suicide at the age of ten. At age thirteen he realized he had a choice and at age fifteen his life changed forever when he read a passage in the Gospel of John. Jesus spoke of a man born blind when he said, "This happened so that the work of God might be displayed in his life" (John 9:3).

Nick is now twenty-eight years old and has traveled to thirty-two countries with his L.A.-based ministry Life Without Limbs. At age nineteen he went into this ministry and started speaking to anyone who would listen to his story. He says, "I can stand in front of the gates of hell and redirect traffic. God asks me every day, 'Do you trust Me?' God says what He means and means what He says." I asked Nick for the traits he'd put on the top of his list for a woman who would be worth dating. Here's what he said:

Everybody has a subconscious list, whether they admit it or not. Mine would include: to love God, to love me, to be called to be my wife, to be a woman of character, to be a meek woman, and be loyal to God. Jesus has to be her rock and everything else will fall into place. When a woman knows who she is in God, then she's at rest. I admire women who love to worship God.

I also want her to know that she's imperfect and so am I. She would have a very independent, relentless love for God. She would be in tune with her femininity. She would be moved by my love. She would see that I am moved by her love. She is gracious. She is calm. She is able to laugh at herself and not take herself too seriously. She is able to enjoy me from across the room when we're not even talking. She is very capable of hearing God.

Jeff is looking for "somebody who communicates mutual respect and support." As a drummer who is on the road a lot, he couldn't promise to be at home all the time. "It's a respect for me as well as my profession. Obviously, she needs to be a Christian and have morals that I respect. Does she have integrity and can I be proud of that? And there has to be a physical attraction."

Here's what Andrew had to say:

I'm looking for virtue; a woman's character is a huge thing. That is central. She needs to be a Christian and have a strong desire to nurture that relationship with God. I want somebody who has heart and passion. Someone who shares a similar understanding of who God is; someone who is on the same page as me. Someone who is in support of the ministry I'd like to be involved in, someone who wholeheartedly endorses my vocation. Someone with whom I can talk about a wide range of topics, someone who is very interested in learning and engaging with the things around them. I actually have a whole list of things I've typed up that I'm looking for.

Cale said, "She has to care about me and my family. She needs to be forgiving because I'm aware of my own imperfections. She should also be an encourager, someone who is behind me all the way in whatever I do. She also should have a sense of humor."

I met two great guys while traveling on the road, Brandon and Bradley Rodermond. Brandon is twenty-one years old and lives in Myrtle Beach, South Carolina. He's the oldest male of eight pastor's kids, who were all homeschooled and blessed to be raised by godly parents. Brandon plays drums and sings. He's in a band with two of his brothers called Beautiful Tension. His brother Micaiah is sixteen and plays keyboards in the band. Their band is enrolled in a leadership training program and partners with churches and youth centers to do outreach events. When I asked Brandon the question "What qualities do you find most attractive in girls you might want to date?" he said, "I've never been on an actual date, but I would say Security! With a capital S! (Not to be confused with pride.) Self-respect and real confidence in who you are goes a whole lot farther than most girls know. Classy ladies who love God, respect themselves, and demand respect from those around them without having to ask for it stand out like a beacon and definitely catch my eye."

His brother Bradley is nineteen years old and lives in the Myrtle Beach area as well. Bradley plays guitar and sings. Besides physical attraction, he said he's looking for "security, maturity, purpose, a love for God...and a good sense of self-worth. She knows who she is, and is not trying to form her identity by finding out what everyone else thinks is cool."

MEETING PEOPLE

Dr. John Gray is the author of the bestseller *Men Are from Mars, Women Are from Venus*. In the follow-up, *Mars and Venus on a Date*, Dr. Gray outlines five stages of dating. Here they are:

1. Attraction
2. Uncertainty
3. Exclusivity
4. Intimacy
5. Engagement

Dr. Gray says, "Moving through the five stages of dating creates the right conditions for you to develop the ability to 'just know' when the right person comes along. It also allows you to 'just know' when you are with the wrong person."[2]

If you're anything like me, fear can get in the way in dating. I sometimes feel like I want to bail before really getting to know someone, simply because it will hurt more if we're further in emotionally and it doesn't work out. My mum said something very wise early on in my dating years. She said that I needed to see through every relationship that had the potential for being "it" until I knew *why* the guy was or wasn't the one for me. Then I could be single with a clear conscience, knowing that I had done everything in my power to develop a relationship that could have led to marriage. I would then know that I hadn't missed the one for me because of fear or not giving someone a chance.

To find the right person, we may have to *be* the right person. And not be afraid to get ourselves out there. When I asked my friend Nathan "What do you think makes a great date?" he said, "Great conversation, either exploring something new together or exploring something that is in common and is very interesting . . .

like her favorite coffee shop. Be confident and be yourself; that is much more attractive than trying to be someone else. Don't be nervous, unless you're really obnoxious."

My friend Justin is twenty-three years old, and has worked as a singer, model, and actor. Regarding his expectations about the first time he meets a girl, he shared, "I like a bit of awkwardness... because you never know what's going to happen. I don't like when a girl gets too dressed up. It sets the tone and can create pressure and expectations." He adds, "A girl who throws out profanity or smokes is a real turnoff for me. I would rather get to know a girl first. I've actually had girls ask for my number without even knowing me."

I asked him what he does when that happens, and he said, "I give them my old phone number. I'm not really lying. This is a phone number for me, just not my *current* one."

Meeting the right kind of people can be a challenge for many single women. Here's a very practical idea from Dr. Henry Cloud. He suggests keeping a log to put you in touch with your traffic patterns and the ruts you might be in... then consider changing your traffic pattern. He says, "The problem is that this traffic pattern is not exposing them to people who are eligible to date. Then when they realize that the log does not show a random occurrence but a fixed pattern, they see the real problem. Real people fall into routines in life: same community, same recreation clubs, same church. That's good, but it doesn't serve dating very well."[3]

BEAUTY IS SKIN—NOT *SKINNY*—DEEP

Andrew and I were talking about what is in the mind of guys when they meet a girl for the first time and think she's beautiful. I asked him to define beauty. Here's what he said: "Beauty is a big concept; it doesn't just deal with physical characteristics. It also gives us a glimpse into our souls and who we are." I've been concerned that too many girls have bought into the cultural obsession with skinniness and think they need to look like runway models. So I decided to ask my friends (you'll hear more of their stories later) for their take on that. Here's a sampling of what they said:

> Don't go for the skinny-minny vibe. It is not attractive to guys! A risk-taking spirit is attractive to me.
>
> —*Julian*

> I like natural-looking girls, a little bit of makeup, but not too much. I think most runway models look like they might break if you gave them a hug. I like some curves.
>
> —*Brendon*

> It is much more of an issue for girls. Guys don't say, 'I want the skinniest girl possible.' Girls can be pretty and not be obsessively skinny. Actually, many times it is not a positive thing for guys to see a girl who is very skinny. An engaging personality is way more important!
>
> —*Robbie*

> Girls worry about the images in magazines and what they see on TV and they compare themselves to that. But in my opinion, there is a great variety in the types of girls that guys are attracted to. I think a girl is obligated to herself and to God to be fit and true to the way God designed her.
>
> —*Stein*

Because of his work in the plastic surgery industry, I asked Nathan, "What do you think the plastic surgery craze has done to women today and how does that affect you as a guy?" He said,

There was a time when plastic surgery was not common; it was a very private luxury that few and far between could afford. It has become a part of pop culture now, and I think has become too common in the Christian culture as well. I think any woman who is dissatisfied with her exterior beauty needs to spend that time focused on being in touch with her inner beauty and her soul. I have watched countless times the cycle begin that says, "But if I changed this, then..."

So many of those women are left with high medical bills and longing for something more; because what was longing for their attention in the beginning was their soul—not external change. As a man, I prefer a woman who is really confident in how she was made, all natural. On the same note, for those who have had plastic surgery, this is not a judgment just an opinion from someone who has seen extremes in this world.

I posted a call on my Facebook and Twitter pages, asking single girls to respond with some questions and comments they'd like for guys to respond to with regard to making first impressions. Here's some of the great stuff I heard.

What is the first thing that you notice about girls you're not interested in?

—*Debra*

The way they carry themselves, such as the way they dress.

—*Robert*

What's one of the *first* things about women that guys key in on when you meet them that does *not* have to do with looks? And what about women do men find to be the most unattractive?

—*Kathryn*

Most attractive—when they care for others and you can see
Christ through them; not attractive—when girls are selfish and
care only about material things.

—*Marcus*

What's one of the most *unattractive* things? There are a few...
women who party and drink it up, women who are not modest
in their appearance. If you walk around showing off your
body, true Christian men will tend to stay away because of the
temptation to look—and it's not a good thing for us. Modest
clothing and dress is always a good thing.

—*Aaron*

Why do guys most generally look on the outside of a girl, but not
at the inside? Why doesn't the heart matter when dating? Don't
guys want to know what kind of heart a woman has?

—*Vickie*

What do you expect on a first date? How can us girls impress
you? What are you looking for?

—*Anna*

FATAL FIRSTS

I asked a few of my friends "What are the fatal mistakes that girls
make on first dates?" Brendon said, "If a guy goes to pay for you,
let him do it. Just be yourself. Even the macho tough guys who put
up a front have insecurities. They are risking rejection as well. Just
know that guys have the same sort of nervousness as you do."

Bradley responded, "When they act way too desperate, needy,
and easy."

Robbie offered some wise advice concerning things that girls do that might scare guys off. He said, "For the average bachelor, there is something that is scary about really committing to someone. A girl that jumps the gun too fast is incredibly off-putting. If the girl takes the leadership, it's not a good thing either. The poets of old understood the power of mystery in relationships." We'll talk more about maintaining some intrigue and mystery in the next chapter. Finally, Shawn said this:

Don't expect the guy to buy the meal ever. Even if you are offended, do not show that. It's presumptuous. Just know that when a guy doesn't pay for the meal, it could very well mean that he doesn't have enough money to pay.

Don't talk too much about yourself. A big part of getting to know someone is listening as much as it is sharing. Don't feel like you need to fill in the blanks. If the guy is comfortable with himself, you won't have to say much. Don't chew with your mouth open. Don't talk about your exes. Don't push the "God talk" too much unnaturally at the beginning. Let it happen organically. Don't feel like the pressure is on to make things happen. You just want to get a sense of the natural chemistry. Don't try to force that, just let it happen.

And, I would add, don't be afraid to be flexible and deviate from the plan. My friend Justin told me this story: "One time a date and I walked into a movie, and it turned out to not be very appropriate, so we looked at each other and said, 'Let's get out of here.' We went back to her place and just played music. It was very relaxed."

EMBARRASSING FIRST DATES

Do you have any embarrassing moments that took place on first dates? If so, you're not alone. Jeff told me his favorite one:

The summer going into my senior year of high school, I was really pursuing a girl who was a high school beauty queen, and she worked at Nordstrom's. I worked third shift and I would go get her breakfast after work and take it to her before she went to work. I was thinking that we would be together our senior year, and this was going to rock. By the end of the summer, the big date opportunity was the Oregon State Fair. We got to the fair. She said, "I love rides," and I said, "So do I!" because I wanted to be cool and not let her think that anything scares me . . . even though I have the weakest equilibrium on the planet and had barfed all over when I was eight years old when my dad took me on the Octopus ride.

Fast-forward ten years, and the first ride that Kim and I went on at the fair was a spinning ride in which the floor dropped out, and we were plastered to the side. We got off the ride and Kim asked, "Are you all right? You're looking kind of pale." I nodded my head that I was fine. We got on another ride that goes around and around. Then she saw *the Octopus*, and we got on it! This was my day of reckoning.

The ride started off and it was cool—we were together, all snuggled up—then it started spinning around. I could no longer contain it, and I just barfed. It got on her lap and her shoes and she was freaking out. I destroyed my shirt. Needless to say, it tainted the rest of the day. I took her home and we told her little brother about the experience. We went back to school the next week and her little brother told the entire freshman class about the experience. I was an assistant with the ninth-grade PE class—and they all knew what had happened! The only redeeming factor of the whole deal was when a ninth grader brought it up to me—that I had puked on Kim—I made the class run laps. Inevitably Kim got nominated to be on the homecoming court our senior year, a new guy came to school that she pursued, and she asked him to escort her. Guess she didn't want to worry about getting puked on at homecoming!

You probably can't top that story (if you can, I want to know about it!), so I encourage you to get out there and be bold—but be yourself. My guy friends said that to me over and over again. You'll never get a second chance to make a first impression. And once you meet a guy you're interested in dating, how do you know what he's really thinking? Is there a magic formula for understanding guys? I don't think so, but there are some things we can learn.

A FEW TAKEAWAYS FOR YOU AND ME

————◦•◦————

- With quality guys, looks are only one component of attraction.

- We cannot let fear rule in dating.

- Don't talk too much. Leave some mystery!

- Don't expect a guy to pay, but let him if he offers.

- Relax and be yourself!

2

Understanding Guys
WHAT ARE THEY THINKING...ABOUT US?

"So give Your servant an understanding heart..."

—1 Kings 3:9, NASB

I used to be a tomboy. I did not like Barbie dolls, I liked Legos! As I grew into womanhood I became a bit more of a girly girl. I'm sure my tomboy phase had a lot to do with having five brothers. I used to play much more with the boys at school than the girls, and for a time I became rather good at foursquare (a game played with a tennis ball and four squares) because I hung out with the boys so much! I always thought I understood guys pretty well. In some ways maybe I do. But in the area of dating, sometimes men can be a mystery.

A friend of mine sent this to me:

If Men Really Ruled the World...

- nodding and grunting would be considered acceptable responses to "I love you,"
- the funniest guy in the office would get to be CEO of the company,

- raises would be tied to the fortunes of your fantasy sports team,
- a "night out with the boys" once a week would be obligatory,
- the workday would start a lot closer to noon,
- tanks would be a lot easier to rent, and
- every anniversary gift you would ever need could be found at the local hardware store.[1]

Do any of these descriptions fit the guys you know? What other things would you add to the list if guys truly ruled the world? The men I know have run the gamut from being the most brilliant I've ever met to being a little clueless...and it's possible that both of those phrases can even describe the same guy at different times in his life. So where do we start in seeking to understand guys? Let's ask a few of them. Here are some of the things I discovered through chatting with my guy friends. Eavesdrop for a while.

FRIENDS FIRST, AN ORGANIC APPROACH

Willie Register is thirty-four years old and lives in San Diego. He has been involved in youth ministry with Young Life and in a few churches and has done some missions work in Uganda and Europe. Recently, he started a company called Youme Clothing, a clothing exchange for people from impoverished countries. He's a pretty unique guy. I asked him about his dating philosophy. He said, "I am very selective. Dating is a very precious thing. I don't think it's healthy to date around because hearts get entwined in emotional ways. I definitely pursue friendships first. God calls us to guard our hearts. When hearts get broken sometimes, we get disillusioned with God. I think it is important to honor God in this way."

This led into a discussion about being friends first. I have sensed that there has been a move away from the traditional model of dating (guy meets girl, guy gets girl's phone number, guy calls girl up and asks her for a date, they go out, then they decide whether or not they want to continue dating). So I decided to ask a bunch of my guy friends their thoughts on this issue. Here's what Willie said in response to the question "Do you think that there is a shift toward a more organic approach to dating today?"

"Yes, and it is a good thing that people are forming genuine friendships. I also think that guys are more afraid to pursue women these days. It is a lot safer for guys. I do think that guys need to step up and come back to a place of pursuing women in an appropriate way. Ultimately, God calls us to take some risks to build our character and make us more like Him."

I continued my discussion with Willie.

REBECCA: How would you encourage women about guys who aren't stepping up?

WILLIE: Don't settle. You are a priceless gift. In Genesis, when God formed woman from man, the Hebrew word used for *made* means "to form into a priceless object." Nothing else in the Garden of Eden could fill the void that Adam had. Too many women today settle for men who do not truly value and cherish them. If you settle, you are enabling men to *not* be who God has called them to be. Trust that God will bring to you what you need.

REBECCA: This can cause girls to go one of three ways:

1. They can become cynical and hard and have an attitude toward guys.

2. They can decide to take it into their own hands and become very forward as the pursuer.
3. They can start dating non-Christian guys.

Girls need to realize that God's got their back and learn to relax in the mission of being God's girl.

WILLIE: Anytime in Scripture God said He was going to do something, He did it. His nature is one of being the Provider. Patience is something we've lost in our culture. A friend of mine encouraged me to look for someone who is running alongside me, not in front of or behind me. And that's what happened when I started hanging out with my girlfriend.

Cale also agrees that we should establish good friendships before starting a dating relationship with someone. He says, "Spending time with girls lets you see how they interact with others, and it makes it more natural."

Here's Nathan's take: "I think it's whatever is going to work for each person. I personally want the one-on-one time and have no problem saying, 'Let's hang out.' The group thing can be nice because it's low risk and there's no pressure."

Here's what Julian Bailey had to say about the whole friendship thing: "I don't think I have approached relationships with girls from the mentality of a dating context... more of a friendship context—it just kind of happens, and it evolves into something, without feeling contrived. I like things to happen organically or naturally." He continues, "I approach dating in a very casual, not heavy way. I think a lot of single people put too much pressure on themselves for certain things to happen—like finding the perfect person and for stuff to happen by a certain time. We've got to be careful not to place burdens on ourselves that God hasn't given us.

If we want to place our faith in God, it would behoove us for our actions to follow what we say we believe."

Quite honestly, I told Julian, "I've been a little afraid to totally let go of this area of my life...at times I've felt that God may not bring the guy I want to marry in *my* timing."

Julian responded, "It's vital that we trust God and wait for His timing and His best. I don't think that necessarily means we should all expect our spouses to fall through the ceiling and into our laps once God decides we've waited long enough. As we meet new people, we're letting God lead us, confident that our steps are being ordered by Him (Psalm 37:23). Whether we're called to be married or to remain single, God has the best in mind for us. I really like this verse in the Bible: 'The blessing of the LORD makes a person rich, and he adds no sorrow with it' (Proverbs 10:22, NLT). God's heart and His character is to bless us, not to burden us."

Stein felt that some guys can pull off the traditional model of dating. He knows a lot of guys that do use the old model: get girls' phone numbers and go out for dinner or whatever. He continued, "Most can't." He said,

There is a book called *The Game*. It is the 'bible' on how to pick up chicks. It's all an act, and it's really bad, and it leaves a wake of girls who have been treated wrongly. I find that in churches women are very guarded. In one church I attended in New York, the guys and girls wouldn't even hang out with each other because they were all afraid of doing something inappropriate and sinning.

I think the friendship model makes the most sense to me today. You can get to know another person in a relaxed setting and use your reason before you get too involved. Dating is not something to be taken lightly.

I asked him, "Then girls shouldn't feel offended if guys aren't following the old dating model?"

He responded, "Dating someone is a risk. When you ask someone to go out you have to wait for her reaction, and it still can be very awkward."

"What if you want to keep someone in the friend zone? How do you navigate it?"

He said, "In my opinion, the only way you can maintain that is if you both come to the same conclusion that there is nothing deeper than just being friends." Then he shared this experience. "I lived in an apartment with three other guys in L.A. Before you knew it, one of the roommates would end up making out with the girl you brought over. After that, it was awkward for everyone involved."

HOW'S A GIRL TO KNOW?

Okay, so we know that the friend zone with the opposite sex is not easy to navigate either. But what do we do if we want something more than to just be friends? How can girls set a guy at ease? How can we give the right signals without being overly flirtatious? Robbie said, "Flirting is a way that girls can show that they are interested in a guy. There are signals that they send. Guys are notorious for not picking up on body language, and flirting is an easy way for girls to tell guys they are interested without directly telling them that they are."

Brendon commented, "A lot of it is nonverbal...laughing and having a good time."

I asked him, "Is confidence attractive or threatening to guys?"

He answered, "I think that part of being secure in yourself is being willing to be vulnerable and show weaknesses. [But] a majority of guys don't want girls to be overly needy. If a guy is confident enough, he can handle a girl who is confident. Some girls can be too confident and can intimidate guys. You don't want a girl who is going to try to 'steal the pants' in the relationship, but you do want a girl who is willing to say, 'Here's what I think...' but still let you be the leader."

Girls do want to respond and be pursued, but it can be tough for girls who are leaders and used to taking charge. Having been in leadership full time since the age of sixteen, I definitely have a fear of being "too much" in a relationship. I had a man I respect once tell me that he feels I "gate my strength" because of this fear. The truth is that the right kind of guy, who is secure in who he is, is not going to be threatened by a strong woman. He will be man enough!

I then asked Brendon, "How can a girl let a guy know she's interested in a God-honoring way?"

He answered, "When a girl is around a guy a lot and gives him a boatload of attention, it seems pretty obvious. For instance, a girl might laugh way more at a corny joke than it warrants—guys pick up on that kind of stuff. Doing nice things, like randomly bringing a guy coffee or visiting him at work, are also ideas for dropping hints. The key is to not smother guys because they need room to pursue."

I talked with Stein about the concern that some girls have about being too manipulative or being perceived as a flirt. How can a girl let a guy know she's interested without being too flirtatious? He answered, "A woman can let a guy know that she likes him by showing interest and listening to him, by engaging him and giving him attention ... then if she has something meaningful to say after listening to him, that speaks hugely to a guy. I think that's the best way. Just be there!"

So what if we want to keep a guy in the friend zone? I asked him, "Do you think it's better that a girl be overt and spell it out with a guy she's not interested in or should she just show it by her actions?"

"If [a guy is] interested in a girl," he said, "neither one is easy to take. Distance by actions is all you need, but if the guy is clueless, you might need to spell it out."

I asked Jeff, "Do you think overt rejection is better than when girls try to give subtle hints that they're not interested?"

"Yes," he said. "Own up to it if you're not *in* the relationship. That's better than dragging it on. Guys are thick-skulled and will have the perception that 'I'm going to change that.' Just come out with it!"

RESPECT IS HUGE

How does a girl show respect to a guy? I was looking for some practical, specific things to pass on to you, and the boys delivered.

Julian said, "By not trying to get the upper hand and dominate. A woman who is disrespectful of herself and tries to be something she is not can actually show disrespect to a guy who is trying to care for and love her—and he feels like what he is doing isn't making a difference."

Jon responded, "A woman [shouldn't] make a guy feel dumb... demean him and put him down. A guy wants to feel like the king of his castle. A guy needs to learn how to be nurturing too. A girl who is overbearing, controlling, and manipulative is insecure. Maybe her father wasn't there for her in this way, and now she's still searching for security."

Robbie's answer? "I don't need a lot of affirmation, but I'm looking more for quality time and loyalty."

Bradley's response: "When a woman pays attention to me and what I'm saying."

Here's what Shawn had to say: "Respect is huge. I need to feel like a woman sees who and what I am and that she respects that. You should never be putting your man down. Even if you feel like he needs to grow, see his true worth and encourage him to grow, rather than belittle or put him down. A man needs to feel like he is succeeding *as a man*."

What kinds of things can girls do to make guys feel respected? Garret offered, "Don't be too pushy and aggressive. If you respond gratefully as the recipient and allow us to lead, then that communicates respect. For instance, one girl I dated put her phone number in my cell phone without me knowing it. At the end of the date, I said, 'It would be great to get your number,' and she said, 'Oh, you already have it.' That *wasn't* the best move on her part."

What kinds of things do girls do that annoy guys? One thing mentioned by Bradley was this: "When girls try to do or say something to constantly keep the attention on themselves."

I asked his brother Brandon what annoys him, and he offered this list:

1. I find it super annoying when girls pretend to be interested in things I like when they're really not—just because they like me. I like it when girls like something different. It means they're individuals and are secure with who they are.
2. When girls act stupid because they think it's cute. It's not. Girls are way more attractive when they act intelligent and mature.
3. When they try to manipulate you by bringing up drama so you will feel bad for them in order to get attention.

I asked Robbie, "Is too much talking from a girl (dominating the conversation) annoying to you?"

And he said, "It can be. I've had some long-distance relationships where we've had to talk for long times without seeing each other. I think it concerns me more what they are chatting about—what I call 'Christian gossip' or whatever—you know, their friends did this and that. For me, intellectual things are very important to talk about."

We continued.

REBECCA: On a date, would you prefer watching a game together or having a romantic dinner?

ROBBIE: It all depends. Both are fun, but I would probably lean toward the dinner, and it depends on what stage the relationship is in. I like business a lot, and I like to talk about it, but I know that it bores about 90 percent of the girls I have dated.

REBECCA: But talking about your interests is one of the ways girls can show you respect.... How do you feel about the culture today in which girls take the role of the pursuer and show interest in a guy first?

ROBBIE: I don't necessarily like it. To some degree I think that emasculates the guy. I think the guy should be the pursuer and should step up and take the lead. Guys are clearly visual, so a girl has to be "in their sight," but not be overbearing.

In response to the respect shown to him from women, Justin said, "I show them respect by opening doors for them, taking them to dinner, paying for them. I like to hang out with them, do fun things, talk to them, and get to know them."

Pretty basic stuff, huh? But sometimes we can make it so complicated.

Some boys are *very* romantic. Here are some things I heard from my guy friends that got a big "aah" from me:

> In this electronic age, we need to take the time to invest in people's lives beyond texting and e-mail. Take out a pen and paper and actually compose a letter to someone. It says that we have taken more time than just hitting Send—and it is a precious gift these days!
>
> —*Andrew*

> One time we flew in a helicopter and went skateboarding. I've also gone to an observatory. It really puts life in perspective and shows us how small we are.
>
> —*Justin*

> If money was no object, I'd fly her to Paris and eat at a sidewalk café.
>
> —*Cale*

> I love writing poetry, so I've been writing poetry for her. I'm going to learn some haiku next.
>
> —*Andrew*

GIVING THEM TIME AND SPACE

One of the things I am hearing from many women is this question: "What am I supposed to do if guys want to lead, but they aren't stepping up?" I asked Stein, "What do you think inhibits guys from stepping up courageously and being proactive in asking girls out?"

He said,

I think it's epidemic. In recent days I think that Christianity has emasculated men. Men are not emboldened to be men as they grow up. It's not the *Wild at Heart* concept. Stay away from sin and stay righteous, which are good things. But the way it is taught does not make a guy courageous about asking a girl out. He has respect for who a girl is in God's eyes but he's afraid that he might screw it up. That's one angle. The reason I might not pursue a girl is that I might think that I have only one shot. So guys might stand back and choose wisely, or be overly cautious—and do nothing. Men are just wusses lots of times. And sometimes spiritual leadership is a problem.

Nathan said the thing that keeps most guys from stepping up is the fear of rejection. He said there is really nothing girls can do to make guys feel safer and less likely to be rejected. "It's not your job. We need to feel confident on our own and be aware of who we are."

I asked Garret, "What scares you most about a deep relationship?"

His response? "Feeling like I'm enough, that I meet a woman's longing and criteria for a godly man."

Similarly, Nathan explained, "It is so important that women know that we are on a spiritual journey, and we need for them to encourage us in that however they can, simply helping us pursue our relationship with God, not necessarily so that they can benefit from it." He continued, "If a guy's interested in pursuing you, and he knows who he is, he will definitely call you back. If you've made it known that you're interested, he'll respond, unless *he's just not that into you!* For guys, being honest about how we feel is extremely vulnerable and can be painful. To give a woman access to our inner lives is very scary. Just know that men think very differently when it comes to tearing down the wall and really sharing who we are. The stake in that is very high."

Jeff adds, "If a guy is interested, he will do anything he possibly can to make you happy. Even if we can't meet all your expectations (like making a boatload of money), we still really want to do our best

---

I CAN'T BE YOUR FRIEND AFTER WE BREAK UP

If you break up with me, you are being unkind by continuing a friendship with me in the immediate period following our breakup. I *want* you to text me, but it would make it much easier if you wouldn't. And please take a couple of months before you date my best friend.

—Matt

---

to genuinely try to make you happy. If you show a grateful attitude toward us, acknowledging our efforts, that goes a long way."

In his book, *Men Are from Mars, Women Are from Venus*, Dr. John Gray says that men are like rubber bands and they need to sometimes pull away before they can draw closer to women, but often women run into their man's cave too quickly and ask, "What did I do wrong?" When I brought this up to Brendon, he responded, "I am wired in a way in which I definitely need my alone time. When you don't have the man cave time, it's easy to feel smothered. If there is no time away, then time spent with a girl is not as refreshing and sweet."

Garret states, "After the first date there is usually a lot of texting and calls. We need more guy time. Girls will leave their best friends to pursue a guy. A guy typically won't do that. We don't want to lose any of our 'guyness.' A girl tends to make a guy 'her world' quickly, and then the guy gets scared because he feels the space closing in. Girls tend to be too persistent."

MORE QUESTIONS THAN ANSWERS

I continued getting some great comments and questions from girls on my Facebook and Twitter sites. I asked them to get creative and personal with it. And they did!

How do I know what to look for when a guy loses interest in me?

—*Lynn*

Do guys like to be the strong one all the time, or is that just a front for pride?

—*Kat*

Why aren't guys man enough to ask the girl out these days?

—*Jillian*

I would like to know why men are afraid to start relationships. Are many men afraid to lead in a relationship? And what can we as women do to make leading easier for them, if anything?

—*Sherri*

Is it true that men between thirty-five and forty-five who are single are reluctant to approach a woman these days because today women pretty much decide what they want? Is this role reversal making more men feel like they should wait for women to approach them? Do they feel if a woman doesn't approach them, then she is not interested?

—*Tina*

Why does it seem that many Christian men do not take as much effort to pursue a woman that they are interested in as in the "old days"? Many women feel like they get mixed signals from men. I have been told that I need to give hints to a man if I am interested, but I believe the role of the man is to take the initiative. It just doesn't make sense!

—*TLC*

Why do you guys not do anything to try and win us beautiful girls? We are not for free!

—*Elle*

Why do guys say they just wanna be friends, then act totally different?

—*Naomi*

Why does a guy date a girl, break up with her, then get back together? What's the point if they're just going to break up again?

—*Marisa*

Why do guys flirt with us if it doesn't mean anything to them?

—*Isabella*

Why is it that sometimes a guy who likes a girl is rude to her and won't admit that he actually likes her?

—*Carolyn*

If a girl's been through trauma, how willing would you be to look past what she's been through and see her heart? (Would you see her as stained?) And how willing would you be to hear her needs and help her to know she can trust you?

—*Janelle*

What are some of the main things girls misunderstand or misjudge about guys?

—*Kelsey*

Are you gonna break my heart or are you in this for the long haul?

—*Sandra*

MYSTERY AND INTRIGUE

Brothers Brandon and Bradley Rodermond named their band Beautiful Tension as a reminder of the beauty of God in His mystery. In their words,

> He is both the Lion and the Lamb, and we can't see a true picture of who He is without a "beautiful tension" between the two. To fully appreciate God's mercy, we must understand His wrath. So often humans choose to experience just one aspect of God and never experience all that He has to offer. For instance, if you have created a picture of a God who is only loving, accepting, and cool with your sin, then you are lacking the fear of God in your life.
>
> God doesn't fit within our boxes. He is entirely otherly! And to truly experience Him we have to take Him for who He is.

I totally agree. So how can we build some of God's mysterious nature into our personalities? A good place to start would be by checking out all the names He's known by in Scripture. Grab a Bible concordance or type "names for God" in a search engine on the Internet. Happy discovering! Just as we are intrigued by the many facets of God, we should create some sense of intrigue for guys in our dating relationships. I asked my friends these questions, "Do you think guys like some mystery?" and "What keeps a guy interested in a girl?" Here's what I heard.

> There is a balance between wanting to be real and open; at the same time, guys want to pursue something that is worth working at. They want a bit of a chase. Don't make it too easy. A little bit of "playing hard to get" is good, but not too much. Show that you have a life apart from the relationship. Don't be so quick to

reply to everything; save a little bit of mystery. Discover your vocation, your individuality. Give the relationship some space. If it's meant to be, then absence really does make the heart grow fonder.

You need to feel like there is something yet to be unveiled, something you can't yet fully enjoy. Ultimately the mystery comes from your relationship with God. Women want to be enjoyed and want to be made to feel like they're beautiful and that they are a prize that has been won.

—*Brendon*

On the topic of mystery, Dr. John Gray says, "When a woman falls in love and behaves as if she is completely won over, as she would in stage five of a relationship, a man will tend to stay in whatever stage he is in. There is no motivation to move ahead. When a woman moves faster through the stages, a man will tend to put on the brakes."[2]

Jon Patton said, "I think a lot of guys like girls who are 'hard to get.' Guys don't want girls to share everything right away. It's a gradual thing. The slower you take it, the more there is to discover."

Julian agrees. He observed, "A woman shouldn't let me in too soon, on all levels. I don't think a girl should show her cards too early or give away that she likes someone too soon. I'm looking for someone who has honor and respect for herself."

Jeff says this is what keeps him intrigued in a relationship: "A woman's own interests that are separate from mine, and if she is really passionate about them! What excites her? Outside of eating dinner and watching movies, what does she do? A guy might say something like this: 'I'm a computer programmer and I come home and watch *Family Guy*...' Is that all there is? A woman of intrigue has much more to offer than that."

SOMETIMES SILENCE IS BEST

I love the TV show *The Office*. The show is pretty much centered around awkward moments between a boss and his office staff. These situations make for some hilariously entertaining television! I started wondering why I could embrace awkward moments on *The Office* but not in my real life. Why couldn't I just inwardly laugh at the strange situations I can get myself into, rather than making them worse by trying so hard to ease the discomfort of awkwardness?

One guy that I dated (we'll name him Sean) asked me to come to Santa Fe, New Mexico, to hang for New Year's with some of his friends and family. As I arrived at his family's home we were greeted by his parents, whom I'd never met before. Sean's dad offered to bring our bags inside, to which Sean said no. They verbally tussled about it for a minute and it became an awkward moment. Trying to make light of the situation I joked, "Now I know where Sean's stubbornness comes from!" Needless to say, no one laughed, and I turned an awkward situation into an even more awkward one!

Sometimes it's best to leave awkward moments as they are and embrace them by letting them go. Even awkward silences with someone we're dating can turn out to be comfortable pauses that allow our date to step into the conversation and lead. Sometimes we girls just talk too much and don't allow our guys to have the space to speak! We can promote mystery by just going with the flow and letting communication happen.

SOME DO'S AND DON'TS

Let's conclude this chapter by asking guys for specific do's and don'ts that girls need to keep in mind when interacting with them.

Here's Brandon's list:

- DO: Communicate, communicate, communicate! Sometimes it feels like guys and girls speak two different languages, so it would be better to share more information than not enough. At least for guys' sakes.
- DON'T: Assume anything; just ask or tell. I think most problems arise when one person in a conflict assumes that the other knows what was done that may have caused hurt. Communication solves misunderstandings before they develop into conflicts.
- DON'T: Get mad about something and keep it to yourself. If something bothers you I want to be sensitive to it, but if you won't communicate, then I don't know how to make it better—or even what the problem was in the first place!

Here's Garret's list:
- DO: Find out more about who I am as a person, about my family, my personal interests, and not just what I do for a living.
- DO: Carry on a good conversation. Ask fun questions like "If you were stranded on a desert isle, what essentials would you have to have?"
- DO: Be honest about your struggles.
- DO: Try to make a guy laugh on the first date. First impressions are huge, and confidence either comes through or not. Sincerity is also very important.
- DON'T: Try to be somebody that you're not.
- DON'T: Try to be too bold.

Here's Bradley's number-one suggestion:
- DO: Be straightforward with guys. Most guys don't seem to read into stuff as deeply as girls and sometimes can't take a hint. If you had fun or if they did something inappropriate or offensive, do us a favor—be up front and let us know.

A FEW TAKEAWAYS FOR YOU AND ME

- Regard dating as something that is precious; don't overdate. God calls us to guard our hearts.

- Keep dating organic and real.

- Foster friendship.

- Don't settle for a man who will not value and cherish you.

- Protect yourself against cynicism toward guys. They can be insecure sometimes too.

- If you want to just stay friends with a guy but he's showing romantic interest in you, be honest with him.

- Flirting (laughing, listening, asking questions, showing interest with your eyes) is a good thing!

- Don't be pushy or dominant. Respond.

- Have a life apart from the relationship.

3

Understanding Us
FLIRTING, BODY IMAGE, AND MAJOR TURNOFFS

"Charm is deceptive, and beauty is fleeting; but a woman who fears the LORD is to be praised."

—Proverbs 31:30, NIV

I once went on a blind date. A former guitar player of mine set us up, and I really trusted his opinion, so I wasn't super nervous as I headed to the café where we were going to meet. Either way, good or bad, I knew I was gonna get a good story out of this little adventure! We met and it was slightly awkward, but not too bad. He was kind, warm, attractive, and he very obviously loved Jesus. The conversation flowed well after we got our coffee; we had a tremendous amount in common. In fact, that was the deal breaker for me. It was like dating myself! At the end of our time together, though it had been a very nice time, I felt no intrigue, no desire to get to know him more. We were simply too similar! Now we did go out one other time; he took me out for a lovely dinner. And he did drop flowers, a teddy bear, and a card by my house for Valentine's that year, but at the end of the day the synopsis was the same for me.

Now, when I look at this story objectively, I feel for guys in their pursuit of understanding us females. Man, have they got their work cut out for them. Yes, we girls can be hard to figure out at times. Here's what a few of my guy friends had to say about their experiences as they have sought to comprehend us—the fairer sex. They had some awesome insights . . .

TRUE BEAUTY

I asked some of my friends for their thoughts on true beauty and femininity. Listen in.

Nathan said, "A woman who is greatly in tune with her 'daughtership' in God, the veil of the bride of Christ, the woman who truly carries grace in her eyes and in her smile is captivated by how God has made her. Therefore, she does not want to change everyone and make them be someone else to make *her* feel better. She feels very soft and loveable in that place. She is content with her own femininity and has received who she is. She lives in that and embraces it."

He continues, "Your femininity is a gift and it is part of the design God made in you. It is meant to be nurtured through the relationship you have with the Creator. So do not measure yourself by your career, the world, TV, or any sort of social media."

My life coach Ken said to me, "Until you own your own beauty you won't offer it to anyone else." It's such a biblical idea—love your neighbor as you love yourself. Own who you are and love who you are—who God has made you to be. It all sounds so easy, but so many women struggle with issues of identity, beauty, and true femininity. If we don't understand ourselves, how can we expect guys to?

I read this somewhere, but don't remember where: "When

From a man's perspective, a woman is most attractive when she is aware of her needs *and* she feels self-assured that her needs will be fulfilled.[1]

I like it when girls are just themselves and they do girly things with other girls—like painting their nails and doing whatever other mysterious things happen when females assemble. Stuff like that seems to refresh them because they're in community like God intended.

—Brendon

A woman is not a piece of meat, she's a flower!

—Jon

a woman appears softer and more feminine, she appeals to [a guy's] instinct to protect; when she appears more aggressive, she appeals to his instinct to compete."

I read that statement to my friend Stein, and he agreed with it. He said, "We want to be stronger, we want the woman to be more feminine. That's how God designed it."

When I asked Andrew what gifts women can bring to a relationship that a guy can't, he responded, "Beauty, compassion, nurturing. The differences that we have should really be highlighted."

I want to be a blessing with my warmth and my softness. I think that our culture tries to knock the softness out of women. I believe that a lack of softness—a hardness—pushes away men. Sometimes we just need to *be*, and not do.

I tend to be a bit of a doer and a pleaser. In one relationship, I remember telling my dad about how the guy was with me and he said, "Bec, it sounds like he just wants to *be* with you...you don't have to *do* or be 'on' all the time because he receives you just the way you are!" I realized that there was such grace that was being shown to me through this guy. I think it's very easy for us to do a lot for the guy with whom we're in a relationship. This is good, but when it becomes about earning approval from a guy, it can be really dangerous. Dating is not about a good performance; it's about being real.

Listen to what Dr. John Gray says: "It is fine to give to a man, but what is great is to receive. The secret to success for a woman in the third stage is to continue receiving. This is the time for her to focus not on doing things for her partner but on receiving. By being receptive and responsive to what a man offers, she is actually giving the relationship the best chance to grow."[2]

Justin concluded, "Girls should be confident in themselves, but still soft. I feel that too many girls try to define themselves by who they are currently with (as though they have to always have a boyfriend). You can't find out who you are or what you want if you are always defining yourself by the guy you are with. You need to know who you are by yourself. Too many girls *need* someone all the time. You shouldn't need someone to fill a void."

A woman who is sure of her inner beauty is confident. Julian said this: "A woman's confidence is appealing. I think one way it is expressed is feeling that you don't have to dress provocatively. It might also be displayed by having an intelligent conversation with me. I like it when someone is willing to challenge me. But I don't like it when someone is always trying to prove that she is right and is constantly wanting to debate. Be confident, but humble."

Nathan said that certain actions reveal that a woman knows who she is and is confident in herself. He pointed out, "A woman exudes confidence by being able to embrace a compliment. And in humility her personality and her actions don't change when you're in the room; she remains the same."

QUIRKY CONFIDENCE

One of the things that I heard over and over from the guys I interviewed is that they love it when a girl is confident in who she is. Owning who we truly are is very attractive to the opposite sex!

My date and I went to Disneyland for the day. I wanted to "kidnap" him and go somewhere as a surprise. So I asked him to keep his eyes closed on the drive there. He had no idea where we were going...until he heard the monorail at Disney! In addition to going on almost all the rides, we watched quite a few street performers and various shows. We talked about the fact that the ones that we enjoyed the most were the shows where the performers brought their own unique personalities to the table. Through humor, facial expressions, and interaction with the crowd, they connected.

Afterward, as I processed this, I realized how powerful it is when we bring our true selves to the table in relationships, rather than hiding behind what we think the other person wants us to be (which I've done way too much) or excusing the parts of us that we might be embarrassed by. What a beautiful gift it is when we come to relationships fully in our own skin—quirks and all.

I'm learning to embrace my quirks. I overpack my travel bag. I swing my arm when I walk. I call a local café my "office." I probably overshare. I like hurdling random things at the mall. I sing songs about the family dog while I'm home in L.A. (he's in Tennessee). To hide these things, though, would be me *not* being me. To the right guy, our quirks are lovable! Girls, let's embrace ourselves so we can offer our full selves in a relationship.

ROLLER-COASTER LOGIC

I love what my friend Cale said when I asked him, "What is the most confusing thing about girls for guys to understand?"

Without batting an eye, he responded, "Women are like roller coasters. They have this incredible draw to them because they are thrilling, but they are incredibly terrifying at the same time!"

From time to time I like going on thrill rides at amusement parks. They're a blast. But have you ever stopped to consider that our emotions sometimes look like that when we're head-over-heels in love? We eagerly anticipate the climb to the top of the hill, then enjoy a fast-paced ride, a loop or two, only to plummet to the depths of despair before we ready ourselves for the next thrilling adventure. There are all kinds of things going on in our minds and bodies. Ups and downs. Pros and cons. Rational thoughts and crazy schemes. And sometimes we decide to bring the guys' emotions along with us for this topsy-turvy ride. Often it's the case that after the experience we each might describe the ride in very different words. We wonder what the guys are thinking, and they wonder what is going on in our minds as well.

I asked my guy friends, "What are some things you wish you understood more about how girls think?"

Bradley answered, "Why certain girls date dirt-ugly guys who treat them poorly, then get upset when nice guys stand up for them and tell their boyfriends to respect them (it may just be the girls in this area, but I don't get it)."

JEFF: Do you want a man who is going to listen to your problems or fix your problems? The answer might be both—but the real question is when? *When* do you want to be listened to and when do you want us to fix it?

REBECCA: I think both are good. I think you should listen until the girl's done venting, then you could ask, "You wanna know what I think?"

JEFF: You just solved all my problems! [pause] Another puzzling thing...why do girls always compare themselves physically to other girls? *(Do my thighs look like that?)* Why is there always a comparison game going on? And why do girls have to constantly question and validate the relationship? That stuff drives us nuts!

Back to Cale. I asked him, "How do you get the feeling that a girl is into you?"

"In my experience," he responded, "they've just told me. Girls can be confusing. Sometimes they send signals and you have to investigate to see if they are legit or not."

Nathan didn't totally agree. He felt like he has a pretty good handle on that. He said, "You can tell by a woman's body language, the smile, the glance. It's obvious. How responsive she is and how inviting she is to more conversation."

My cousin Matt talks about what he calls the "I want to be pursued" phenomenon.

Christian girls have strange expectations of what a guy should do in a dating scenario. They all want to be pursued, but they are also very cautious about showing interest in a guy—even if the girl really likes him. I get it. I really do. Dating is a game of cat and mouse. However, at some point a girl needs to take a chance and respond.

Girls often expect a guy to keep pursuing them even though they have responded to the guy's advances with *nothing at all*. That is an unfair power play, and ultimately flawed understanding on how a guy thinks and what he can handle. No man is bulletproof. It takes two to tango and at some point you are going to have to take a chance on a guy and see if you can dance.

When I asked Garret about things guys don't understand about girls, he said, "I think girls often don't allow the relationship to be easy. Why do they make it so complicated? They make it more complex than it has to be. Why do they have to read into everything too quickly? (Just because I didn't respond immediately to a text doesn't mean I was talking with another girl!) Many girls are jaded because they've been treated badly in past relationships."

I've known people who have had several hurtful things happen in past relationships, and they've decided it is no longer worth trying. That's unfortunate. Part of the risk of loving is the risk that you *will* get hurt. But we must realize that the potential pain is worth it.

Garret cautions, "Don't box a guy into being 'like the guy before.' Don't put a stigma on him right off the bat. You have to trust him and not peg him to be like previous guys. Give him a chance. Come into a relationship with an open mind and a guarded heart."

I have done exactly that before. When I explained to my boyfriend at the time that my actions had been based on some of my past experiences with other guys, he said, "But I am not those 'other guys.'" It was a healthy reminder for me not to live in fear.

WHAT ARE YOU LOOKING FOR?

Facebook brought to the surface some other interesting comments and questions. Here's a sampling.

Are guys intimidated by athletic girls? (I play basketball.) What are your thoughts on shyness vs. being outgoing? When I'm quiet, guys tell me that I scare them, but I feel loud and annoying when I'm outgoing. Can you help me understand?

—*Patricia*

Do you think that you should establish a good friendship with a girl before beginning a dating relationship?

—Pretty in Pink

Why do you guys let the nice, quiet girl sit on the sidelines while you make a fool of yourselves for the girl in the miniskirt?

—Fransisca

Why do guys fall for the girls that flirt with everyone?

—Lauren

What is the first thing that makes you notice a girl? 'Cuz I need to figure out what I need to work on.

—Samantha

I would like to know what guys look for in a girl. Do they have high standards? Why don't some guys just accept us the way we are?

—Amber

I just met a lady who was interested in and talked about business, finance, and serving others. We talked for hours last night. A spontaneous connection like that will touch your heart.

—Jeremy

From a Christian man's perspective, a girl should find three things in a Christian guy before they enter courtship: 1. he is set with his career (he has to be ready to provide); 2. he has a car ('nuff said); and 3. he has a house ready for you to fill. Don't accept anything less.

—Derek

Derek, God can provide those things in the midst of courtship.
I have a friend who had just that experience. He had a car and
career from the start and was able to obtain his own place
readily. But it just seems too shallow and missing some important
points to set those as preliminary requirements before a girl gets
to know a guy. We can't live by practicality alone.

—*Matt*

What do guys think about girls who pursue them? I was taught
to be pursued by the guy.

—*Monique*

Is it okay if girls ask the guy out or is that socially incorrect?

—*Maribeth*

TOO MUCH PRESSURE

According to the *New York Times*, the number of single women
in America has exceeded the number of married women. Only 49
percent of women are now married and living with a spouse (53
percent of men).[3]

This article goes on to state, "In 2005, married couples became
a minority of all American households for the first time." I have
to wonder if that is why so many single women I know feel the
urgency to get married. That can create lots of undue pressure on
themselves as well as on the guys in their lives. I asked guys in
what ways they have felt pressured by women. Here's what they
said.

There is an understanding that the man should be the head of
household, the provider. There can be a lot of pressure that goes

with that. I would encourage you to try and focus more on the guy's efforts and his character.

—Shawn

There is so much pressure to be more than friends. If a girl gets too serious too early, and she becomes impulsive, it scares me.

—Justin

Some women can be too aggressive, too feisty. They might give you a hard time based on what you are wearing or what you said. They might be pugnacious and just want to debate you. Aggressive, controlling behavior invokes a man's competitive nature—it's really a pride issue.

—Stein

Females need to talk; that's how they emote, that's how they connect, but sometimes they apply pressure by talking too much. Guys just have to accept that. Usually, girls don't want us to tell them how to solve it; they don't want a solution, they just want to emote and have us listen.

—Jeff

Is there anyone out there who wonders if God has purposed the population this way for a reason? Why are there so many more single women than there are single men in my age bracket [thirty-five to fifty years of age]? There are 28 percent more women on this planet. Has God purposed us to be single for a reason, for His use?

—Elaine, on Facebook

Some guys feel serious financial pressure. I asked a few of my friends what they thought about dating or marrying someone who makes more money than they do, or is more successful in their career. I asked if that would intimidate them. Brendon said, "I don't think it's that big of a deal, unless there's a huge disparity. There's nothing in the Bible that says the guy needs to make more money. He can still lead."

Nathan laughed and responded, "I say the more bacon she brings home, the merrier! Seriously, what's most important to me is that she is doing something that she is really passionate about, regardless of how much money she makes."

MAJOR TURNOFFS

When it comes to understanding girls, what are the typical things we do that drive guys crazy? I asked the boys about high-maintenance girls and other turnoffs. Here's what they had to share.

"Being high-maintenance means being insecure, always making me explain why I did such and such or said something to someone or looked at them a certain way," Julian said. "It comes back to disrespecting a guy. That will wear you down, and it's just not enjoyable."

Nathan responded, "A high-maintenance woman constantly talks about herself. She has such a deep need and longing to connect that she can't see past her desperation, so she spends too much time overcompensating and defending who she is. It's not very enjoyable to be around someone like that. All you see is the insecurity and the level of maintenance she requires."

Cale said, "If women are really awkward and can't carry on a conversation, then that's a problem."

Jeff observed, "A girl shows her insecurity by always looking

---

TOP TEN TURNOFFS FOR GUYS
(IN NO PARTICULAR ORDER)

1. A critical spirit, not being gracious in the relationship.
2. A hot girl who is boring.
3. Someone who doesn't know how to have fun.
4. The inability to be feminine (wear some high heels every now and then!).
5. Constant texting and e-mailing (please give us some space!).
6. Girls who show too much skin; they're saying, "all I'm worth is my body."
7. Girls who worry too much about how they look.
8. Girls who don't worry enough about how they look.
9. Jealousy.
10. Smoking.

---

for affirmation. An insecure person is never going to be fully happy."

Stein shared about the things that are turnoffs for him.

Girls worry too much about how they look. If a woman won't ever let you see her without her makeup, then it says something about a lack of confidence.... On the other extreme, there are the girls who are afraid to look hot. Optimize the physical—in a godly way! Some girls, for whatever reason, are not free to be feminine. They're always wearing jeans, a sweatshirt, and gym shoes. That's fine, but every now and then they need to break out and wear the red dress and high heels, and feel better about themselves.

For Brandon, a big turnoff is "when girls only act sweet or nice to guys they think are cute, but act jerky to other girls or guys that they don't think are attractive. I like girls who are legitimately sweet people, not just able to turn it on when they want to flirt."

Big turnoffs for Bradley? "Tattoos, flirtiness, cussing (some girls think it makes them look so cute, but it's just not classy and it says that they don't respect themselves or the people around them), and smoking! Nobody wants to kiss an ashtray!"

Julian is turned off by "someone who has a rebellious heart toward God, someone who is overly independent, someone who is domineering or overbearing, someone who smothers and suffocates others. I prefer a girl who has her own thing going on."

Cale said that the biggest turnoffs he's seen include "girls who are really attractive, but who are really self-centered. When all they talk about are the things they have done that week, they stop being interesting. Really controlling girls are also a turnoff. Let the guy be the guy and the girl be the girl!"

IT'S HARD WORK

A friend told me about a dating book she had just read. I love to read, so I asked her more about it. As she shared I had an instant dislike of the title, *Marry Him: The Case for Settling for Mr. Good Enough*.

Ouch. That just sounds wrong, doesn't it? We're not meant to settle! We're meant to hold out for Mr. Right! We're not meant to marry because of the fear of being left on the shelf; we're meant to wait as long as it takes for the magical relationship! Well, I ended up reading the book, partly to research for the book you are reading right now and partly because my curiosity got to me. The book is actually a wonderful read, one I would thoroughly recommend for anyone twenty-five years old and above. Sometimes we believe too much in the fairy tale that movies and books promote and we feel that it needs to come true in our own lives. But life is not a fairy tale. And there is a place for our dreams to be tempered with wisdom, truth, and reality.

"People don't expect to work in relationships today.... I think a lot of women nowadays expect that they'll always get every single one of their needs met and if they don't, something's wrong. Nothing's wrong—that's just the nature of two people being in a relationship."[4]

My parents have continually told me that marriage is hard work but completely worth it and one of God's greatest gifts. In my experience, at times dating seems to be similarly difficult. Hard work... but worth it.

Ready to talk about getting spiritual in our relationships? Turn the page.

A FEW TAKEAWAYS FOR YOU AND ME

- As God's daughter, own your unique beauty and femininity.

- *Be* in a relationship with a man. Try *doing* less. Learn how to receive.

- Stay soft.

- Don't compare yourself to other girls.

- The possibility that you might make more money is not necessarily a problem for your guy.

- Don't read into everything. Try not to make things complicated.

- We often show our insecurity by constantly looking for affirmation.

- Good relationships take WORK!

4

Spiritually Connecting

GOD AND GUYS

"Let us fix our eyes on Jesus, the author and perfecter of our faith..."

—Hebrews 12:2, NIV

For years I've been bringing the eighties back by rollerblading my little heart out at the beach where I live in California. Awhile back I was out in the sunshine going for a long rollerblade. And I was lost in my thoughts. Thinking about a boy. Dissecting every detail of my relationship with said boy. About halfway through my ride I felt the Holy Spirit gently nudge me, "Rebecca, look up." I realized that I had been staring at the ground as I bladed, worrying, analyzing my dating life, not looking up and around, and—most of all—not looking for God to speak to my situation. I realized that I wasn't awake to a few very necessary things.

Awake to the fact that I could trust God to take care of me, that I didn't have to worry or be anxious.

Awake to His beauty around me, evoking worship.

Awake to the lives and needs of others around me.

I think it's very easy for us girls to get so caught up in

relationships that we become blind to the other things that are going on around us. The spiritual dimension of a relationship is very important. Here's what I discovered about how guys feel about their walk with God and how it relates to the girls they pursue.

HONORING GOD TOGETHER

Brothers Brandon and Bradley Rodermond shared some really cool information with me regarding their upbringing. My friends have the floor.

Growing up in a big family has taught us how to lead, work hard, show grace to others, and appreciate diversity. Through preparing meals, doing laundry, and getting out of the house on time, multitasking has become a way of life. Most importantly, we have learned from firsthand experience that there is no room for pride and selfishness in our lives.

God continually reminds us of our need to rely on Him and the people He puts in our lives—for everything. God has given us a passion for Him, and to see His kingdom advanced. Our parents passed on not only a love for God, but also a heart for ministry. They did it by teaching us to serve others—by cleaning churches, setting up chairs, making coffee (and cleaning up coffee stains from the church carpet), teaching kids' church, working nursery, scrubbing toilets, and anything else that needed doing. As we started playing music, we learned to use our talents for God by playing and singing with the worship team as well as by leading the youth worship. Eventually, we felt prompted by God to record some of the songs He had given us, so we began building a tiny makeshift home recording studio in our bedroom. We knew absolutely nothing about recording music, and had very limited technology to work with, but still we felt God's beckoning and pressed on. From recording to mixing tracks to mastering—and overcoming hurdles all along the way—God proved himself faithful in leading us step by step. The most important step we took was dedicating each and every song to God, while saturating them in prayer and worship.

This attitude of servanthood, humility, and unity is so important in the ministry, in our homes, and in our relationships. As we move deeper into the stages of dating, it is key that we work hard at developing the spiritual aspect. Physical and emotional chemistry is very important, but without the spiritual, we cannot walk in the kind of relationships to which God has called us.

What does it mean to honor God in a relationship? For Brandon it means "to pursue God first. . . . If God is the center of the relationship, in pursuing Him we grow closer together. It also means that we must set forth biblically based boundaries and standards from the very beginning of the relationship. That way, when temptation arises there is already a clear line drawn."

Bradley adds, "It means that we put Him first, and live by *His* standards that He outlined in Scripture for our own good, rather than by what we *think* we can handle."

Andrew explains, "Realize that the other person is a son or daughter of God, so we should treat them with respect. Women are precious and should be treated with love and care."

Julian put it this way: "Guys and girls should respect each other physically by not crossing any lines or by testing any boundaries. Before any gray area appears, boundaries (concerning what we think is okay, and what we believe God is asking of us) should be established. Treat each other with integrity, and don't lead one another on if the relationship is not heading toward marriage."

Stein got a little more specific:

You honor God by being pure because your body is His temple. When you engage in inappropriate sexual relations you do something extraordinarily defiling. It's worse than anything else because it possesses the mind. Don't let lust ever come into it and don't let yourself be overcome with the easiest possession that you could ever have. Girls, you honor God by not dressing too sexy and by keeping God as the center of your relationship. When you fall in love, this person becomes larger than life and can definitely become an idol.

Garret responded, "You honor God by the way you treat each other—with honor, dignity, and respect. If we're not careful, the physical attraction can take over the core. If that happens, then God is no longer the core of the relationship. You have to keep God in the center of it, by being more intentional about praying about the relationship."

Nathan agrees, "Prayer is a huge part of it. I need to have clarity on what it means to honor God by spending individual time with God. Whether or not a woman will be my lifetime partner I still should treat her with the utmost respect, encouraging her and not doing anything that would put her in a position of vulnerability. I also honor God and her by letting her remain whole in who she is."

My friend Willie shared his story with me:

I am black, and the girl I like right now is Korean. But it's been a struggle because of some cultural prejudice. We feel like God has called us to this relationship, but at the same time we want to honor her parents. Our desire is to honor the Lord and obey Him first and foremost. If God is in this and He wants us to be together, then we are going to follow Him into this relationship; and if God says it's time to be done, then we'll break up and we'll walk away. Ultimately, we want to do what *God* wants us to do.

And, ultimately, that is what it means to honor God in our relationships.

PRACTICAL WAYS TO KEEP A SPIRITUAL FOCUS

My mum and dad have a beautiful relationship that I admire very much. Dad had this to say about the spiritual element: "Prayer challenges any tension that might be lingering in a relationship."

I wanted the guys to answer this question, "What good ways have you discovered that help maintain a spiritual focus in a relationship with a girl?"

Brandon's answer? "Having someone that you're accountable to (other than the person you are dating) who can tell you when your focus has shifted from God to the other person. God should always be number one, especially when you are pursuing marriage."

Cale said, "Some couples read the Bible together and then discuss it. Ask mentors who know you both well for some advice and accountability."

Garret shared, "With one girl that I dated we exchanged Bible verses from time to time. I would share a verse that really meant a lot to me, then she shared one that meant a great deal to her. Then we would focus on these verses for a week or so. It was one of the things that made that relationship very special."

Brendon challenges us with these thoughts:

God is eternal and faithful and will never let you down, but guys will. Put your trust in God, not in the guy you're dating. If your value is in only the guy, you are setting yourself up to be crushed.

Some practical ways to honor God in your relationship include being in the Word—have something you can discuss that God is teaching each of you. Learn from each other. I pray with my girlfriend before we eat meals together, but I try to be careful about praying too intimately with her. I've heard some people say that couples should not pray together because of how intimate it can make the relationship too early.

Another thing is serving together. You learn about people by serving together.

Willie continues with his story: "My girlfriend and I are reading *Experiencing God Day by Day* together, and we're also reading through the Bible book by book, so that the foundation of our relationship is the Word. We also pray together on the phone or over Skype (since we live in different cities), and we've seen God bind our hearts together on various decisions.

"We've pursued the Lord together, and have sought to keep Jesus central in our relationship. We have attended church together, but have also given space to pursue the Lord individually."

Blaine Bartel has said, "The world's idea of dating is dangerous at best.... We renew our minds with the knowledge of God's Word. Here are three ways a Christian dating experience should be different from one in the world."

1. In the world, people date to check someone out; a Christian date is focused on building someone up. A Christian's focus should be on encouraging each other in life and in one another's walk with God.
2. The world bases a large part of success in their dates on connecting physically, while Christians should be prizing spiritual things first.
3. The world will often lie and deceive to achieve their goals in dating. Christians are to be committed to integrity and honesty.[1]

EYES ON JESUS

Recently I went out on the balcony to watch the sunset, and had a major moment with God. God speaks to me a lot through nature and through visual pictures. The sky was beautiful—lit up with pink, orange, and purple clouds, tinted by the retreating sun. I watched as some of the clouds lowered beneath the horizon and turned gray. No longer being touched by the sun's rays, they became colorless. But the ones that could still *see* the sun remained radiant. I felt God remind me that as long as I am looking to Him I too will be full of life and color. King David said, "Those who look to Him are radiant" (Psalm 34:5).

But when I'm not looking at Him, because of sin, worry, or fear getting in the way—or because I'm too focused on a guy—my light dims. I fade to gray.

INDIVIDUAL INDEPENDENCE

I believe that we can't get from someone else what we can only get from God. I think a lot of women are looking for a sense of security from men, even though they should be looking for this from God. He alone provides true security, a positive self-identity, and unconditional love—among other things.

Shawn Thomas agrees. He says, "We need a true understanding of how our identity with God impacts our relationships. If we can't love God first, then we really can't love our neighbors as ourselves. All of our relationships must align with this priority."

I asked Nick how important self-respect (which should be coming from God) is to women. He answered,

> It's not how you look or how smart you are, not anything that the world says. It's who you are in the mirror of the Word. If you are

grounded and rooted in the character of God, then you become like-minded with Christ. Your self-respect comes from knowing who you are in Christ and honoring Him. Every breath that you breathe is a gift. Respect yourself to the point that you don't need to change one thing. You are not your own, you belong to God.

Brandon agreed that men and women should be dependent on God, not each other, for our identities. He challenges us, "Don't plan your quiet times with God solely with the other person. Pursue God on your own time, as well as together. Look to the Scriptures daily to reaffirm your identity—who you are in Christ—and God's opinion of you."

I asked Brendon, "Do you think a lot of girls try to find their identity and validation in a relationship with a guy?"

YOUR IDENTITY

You are human (Genesis 1:26).
You are God's masterpiece (Ephesians 2:10).
You are imperfect (Romans 3:23).
You are righteous (2 Corinthians 5:21).
You are chosen (1 Peter 2:9).
You are free (Galatians 5:1).
You are loved (John 3:16).
You are a saint (Ephesians 3:17–18).
You are extraordinary (1 Peter 2:11).
You are indispensable (1 Corinthians 12:22).
You are a child of God (Romans 8:15–17).
You are a priest (Revelation 1:5–6).
You are an overcomer (Revelation 12:10–11).[2]

BRENDON: Yes, especially because of so many father/daughter broken relationships. They should find their identity in Christ, not in a guy. A girl should be saying, "I'm the daughter of God, and this is what I deserve, and I'm not going to settle for anything less."

REBECCA: What other advice would you give girls who are trying to find their validation anywhere other than from God?

BRENDON: You're never going to be satisfied if you try to find your validation in a guy. That puts a lot of pressure on guys to be something they can't be. And it pushes guys away.

I asked Justin and Garret, "What is it about a girl who loves God that makes her unique?"

Justin answered, "Because I'm a Christian, I'm looking for a girl who loves God, is trying to stay pure, and is going to push me spiritually. She will be someone I can trust. If she's chasing after God, and so am I, then as we both draw closer to God, we'll draw closer to each other."

Garret stressed, "By embracing her relationship with God and pursuing Him wholeheartedly with reckless abandon, a girl shows she is serious. If her guy is pursuing God on his own, the bond they share together is very powerful and much more intimate."

FACE TO FACE WITH GOD VIA FACEBOOK

If I were to start a relationship with you, would it lead me closer to God or would it cause me to drift farther away from him?

—*Nancy*

A woman's heart should be hidden in God, so that a man has to seek Him first to find her.

—*Andrea*

I think the first question is "do you love the Lord?" And if he does, find out how he shows it or even ask how he shows it. A man that genuinely loves the Lord above all things would be a great spiritual leader, boyfriend, husband, etc. When I was dating my wife, the first thing I noticed was how she loves the Lord and how she shows that love in worship. I think this suggestion works both ways; girls can ask that question and guys can also.

—Edward

Where are all the men who love the Lord?

—Christina

It just seems like all the Christian guys around here are either taken or just nonexistent. I would like to know, where are they hiding?

—Ainslie

Don't try to impress guys. The wrong guys will want ungodly things and they're still not impressed. Godly men want to see a pure heart. Just be true to God. That's what really matters.

—Brian

Be each other's best friends! Let your guy wait for the first big kiss; this way you will see if he is really interested in you or your body.

—Gregg

Thanks very much for boosting my hope, Brian. I guess I just have to keep on looking out for the right guy while patiently praying without ceasing or complaining. I am encouraged by your stance and belief.

—Cindy

I wanna know: "How well can you handle life situations?"
"Do you respect and treat your mother well?" "Are you seeking
God?"

—*Silvia*

I was wondering what guys thought of girls dating God and
skipping dating altogether (just having guy friends and working
on *their own* character till they find the right guy and God gives
the okay).

—*Dede*

A HEALTHY RELATIONSHIP

I asked several guys, "What does a healthy relationship look like
to you?"

CALE: It's one that puts Christ at the center.... I think that's
hard to do.

BRADLEY: One where both individuals look to God first and
foremost for acceptance and validation, then to the other
person.

BRANDON: It looks like my parents. They have been married
for twenty-six years and love each other just as much now as
the day they got married. They are living proof that it can be
done.

JEFF: One that exhibits grace, humility, and forgiveness. Two
people should be able to come together and say, "You be you
and I'll be me." We'll learn about each other authentically.

That kind of attitude establishes trust in a relationship. A man
and a woman should both be willing to "give preference to one
another in honor" (Romans 12:10, NASB)...to *outdo* one another

with love. I want someone who is passionate about God because I want him to be getting his cues about how to love me from God. We shouldn't be living to just get by, or just to try and fill a void. We should be living for a much higher purpose. We should be learning to love one another.

I'd like to close this chapter by sharing a very cool conversation I had with my friend Nick Vujucic about the spiritual dimension of relationships. Pull up a chair and listen in.

REBECCA: When you think of a person you are dating as your brother or sister in Christ, it creates a whole different focus on the relationship, doesn't it?

NICK: Relationships are about giving, not just about sharing and receiving. In my limited experience, I've seen that it's all about giving.

REBECCA: Our purpose in dating and in marriage should be about how we can help them grow more in their walk with Jesus, how we can help further their growth and help them pursue holiness. How can I bless, how can I serve, how can I give? How has God aligned our lives? . . . Every relationship involves risk. God wants us to just open up our clinched fingers and open our hands to Him, and trust Him, rather than just trying to cling and hold on and try to figure it all out on our own. . . . How do you know if you are in love?

NICK: The first thing is attraction, both inside and out; second is infatuation; and third is getting to know a person's character. It takes time to organically grow into a friendship. . . . (I've had a lot more crushes than being in love. Now I'm very cautious, because I know how easily I can get emotionally attached.) Fourth, there's an emotional and spiritual connection. Being in love with someone would mean that our spirits are attracted to each other. At every step we must pray to make sure it is from God. God will guide you according to His will if you will pray *for* His will.

REBECCA: When you love someone you want to see them be all that they can be, joyful and happy and full—and you want to be a part of that fullness in their life. There should be a soul connection and understanding that is deep and profound. There is a trust and depth that is incredibly unique to that person. There is a strong physical attraction, but there is also a way in which you further one another spiritually, and you can see yourself growing old with this person because they bring out the best in you. There is a different lens through which you can view life because of this person. The final element is that you let go of your inhibitions emotionally. There is a gate that opens in your heart. That's why Solomon cautions three times not to "awaken love until the time is right" (Song of Solomon 2:7; 3:5; 8:4, NLT).

So now that we've set a spiritual tone for what should be happening in our relationships, let's talk about the physical aspect. You thought I'd never get there, huh?

A FEW TAKEAWAYS FOR YOU AND ME

- Look to God and surrender your dating life to Him.

- Realize that the person you're dating is God's son; treat him with respect.

- Honor God by dressing in a pure way.

- Keep God at the center of your relationship.

- Pray.

- Put your trust in God, not in the guy you're dating.

- Be on a mission; serve others and each other.

5

Physically Connecting
MODESTY, SEXUALITY, AND BOUNDARIES

"Run from sexual sin! No other sin so clearly affects the body as this one does. For sexual immorality is a sin against your own body."

—1 Corinthians 6:18, NLT

I was sitting in the car with a guy right outside his house. He got out of the car, went inside, and came back with freshly cleaned teeth and minty-fresh breath. Curious, I asked him why he had brushed his teeth. Ah, the naiveté of a girl who had never been kissed! I figured it out later.

When we were talking about the "physical stuff" for this chapter, my cousin Matt said something very inspiring to me: "The longer it takes for a guy to kiss a girl, the more intrigued with her he becomes." Yet I heard from some of the guys I interviewed how very *forward* many girls are these days—sometimes even more so than the guys! Why is that?

Matt continued, "Guys notice all physical touch signals. Girls need to know this: I realize that I'm meant to be the leader, but the more physical you are with me, the harder it is for me to stop.

Please know that if you touch my arm during a movie or just to get my attention, I am going to think that you are keen." I don't think he means the word *keen* in the sense of "smart."

God desires that His daughters be smart, pure, holy, and set apart from the world. Walking in purity of mind and body—being singularly focused on who God has called us to be—is not old-fashioned or prudish; it is something that is exciting, passionate, and creative. Maintaining mystery and intrigue and not "showing all the goods" is quite attractive to the kind of man you should be seeking for your future husband. The guy who wants to wait for that and experience that with you—and you alone—in marriage is a guy worth waiting for.

Yet I see many Christians these days looking for loopholes, trying to see how far they can go without really getting themselves in trouble. This area of our lives is so important to our worth, to our future, and to our future spouses. Is it possible to find a guy these days who has kept himself sexually pure? Absolutely. I talked with several guys who have committed to waiting for their future wives. Guys like Brandon Rodermond.

Brandon said, "I have kept myself pure as a gift to my future wife, as well as to honor God. I look forward to giving my whole heart to the person I will spend the rest of my life with."

Cale remarked, "It's really black and white in the Bible; it would be awkward to have to tell a future spouse that you didn't save sex for them. I wouldn't want to be in that position with my future wife."

I'm encouraged when I hear people like Cale share their passion for purity. I hear many girls ask, "Where have all the good guys gone?", implying that they see a lack of guys with strong morals and standards. The young men in this book definitely represent the fact that there are a bunch of guys out there with a heart to honor God and women in relationships. And there are also many guys

> God wants you to live a pure life.
>
> Keep yourselves from sexual promiscuity.
>
> Learn to appreciate and give dignity to your body, not abusing it, as is so common among those who know nothing of God.
>
> Don't run roughshod over the concerns of your brothers and sisters. Their concerns are God's concerns, and he will take care of them. We've warned you about this before. God hasn't invited us into a disorderly, unkempt life but into something holy and beautiful—as beautiful on the inside as the outside.
>
> If you disregard this advice, you're not offending your neighbors; you're rejecting God, who is making you a gift of his Holy Spirit.
>
> —*1 Thessalonians 4:3–8,* The Message

who have made mistakes in the area of sex but have been forgiven of their past and are now committed to living in purity. Praise God for His grace toward all of us!

AWAKENING LOVE

I asked, "Why do you think so many Christians are trying to find loopholes in the command to stay sexually pure until marriage?"

Nathan explained, "Because the pressure has been so intense. Sex is everywhere—it's on car commercials, it's on toothpaste commercials....Sex has not been talked about enough in the church in regard to what an incredible gift it is, how powerful it is, how intimate it is. Because people are physically charged, it's all about the physical when you're fresh out of high school and people don't realize how much work goes into creating that kind of intimacy." He continued, "Sex is the strongest link to intimacy without having to be emotionally intimate. It's the easy default to true intimacy."

Jeff replied,

Because we've seen many other Christians give in to it, it becomes easier to justify it. We tend to think, "Well, *he's* a Christian and he's doing it; I guess it's not that bad!" If everyone's drinking at a party, then it's much easier to succumb to that! Unfortunately, we don't live in a society where people applaud personal integrity and strength and leadership. It's just a follower nation in which people go with the flow—don't rock the boat and make it as easy as possible to blend in. There are more insecure people in the world than there are secure people. And because of their insecurities they will try to find fulfillment in sexual activity, and they justify it by thinking about how many other people have done the same thing. Afterward, they may feel like garbage, but who do they go to for empathy? People who have experienced the same thing!

When they really want to make a change, they go to people who aren't involved in sexual activity to see what's different. Then they ask, "Why are they happy? What do I need to do to find true happiness?" There is so much pressure to fit in that people are willing to do things to be accepted. The scariest thing for most people is to be alone and not feel like you are a part of something.

Stein observed, "Girls are so eager to fall in love; sometimes they get really lonely and they don't use their instinctive walls to filter out the bad men. So many guys are relentless that eventually girls give in and they end up with bad guys. I say to girls: be leery, because a lot of guys are creepy...listen to the discernment that God gives you."

Justin pointed out that there are consequences of going along with the crowd in the area of sexual promiscuity—beyond the obvious physical risks of sexual disease. He said, "I think that's why the divorce rate is so high—too many people built their dating relationship on the physical, then had nothing deeper to fall back on when the other person became boring."

Stein shared these thoughts:

You can awaken love far too easily. Falling in love has more to do with how physical you get with somebody than people give it credit for. Ideal dating is not getting to second base or third base (and certainly not having sex). It's taking it slowly and treating each other with respect—and you do that by getting to know one another. Spend quality time with your *pants on*. Once you start making out (on the couch or in a car) people get so dumb, and it taints everything—it permeates the whole relationship—and you get ahead of reason. Set your standards and ideals ahead of time.

Robbie offered, "A lot of it comes down to the influence of the media in our lives. We are inundated with more sexual material than ever. What you watch and listen to is so critical to maintaining your purity. It's so important to see role models who have 'made it' and remained pure."

A pure, unashamed godly sexuality is the most powerful thing in the world. It's very liberating. There's no guilt and no condemnation, and there are no horrible feelings afterward. It's true freedom in Christ.

SETTING PHYSICAL BOUNDARIES

In 2008 I wrote a book entitled, *Pure: A 90-Day Devotional for the Mind, the Body and the Spirit.* I addressed the various aspects of striving after purity—in our thoughts, in our actions, and in our soul. I really believe that one of the important keys in maintaining sexual purity in relationships with guys is to set clear physical boundaries before we go farther than we really want to. On day thirty-eight of that devotional, I shared these words:

I feel that we women have a responsibility not to tempt our brothers in Christ. We really need to help them out in the lust department. We need to be careful and be wise in the clothes choices we make. I have set certain boundaries for myself in the way that I dress. It can be a real challenge at times to find things that are modern and funky and 'today' but still have an element of modesty. I try to take advantage of the unique locations I get to visit. Europe has great clothes—and I love to shop there.

"How far is too far?" If our goal is to honor God with our bodies, then we will draw the line and ask God for the strength not to cross it. One basic principle I live by and often share with others is to not let a guy touch them in any area that a swimsuit would cover. That goes for touching guys as well. A good question to ask is always, "If I participate in this activity, will I have a hard time explaining to my future spouse what I did with someone else?"[1]

Besides the "swimsuit principle" referenced above, some of my other physical boundaries included not taking my clothes off, not being alone with a guy in a bedroom with the door shut, and not lying down on a bed together. I was hanging out with a guy I was dating once and he noticed that I avoided lying on the bed together. I explained to him that I felt that there's something sacred about the bed (Hebrews 13:4). I told him that I want my first time to lie on a bed with a guy to be on my wedding night. He loved it and really respected that I was keeping this as a special gift! I want to live above reproach.

As I talked with my guy friends, I asked them, "How can girls help guys set and keep physical boundaries?" Here's what they offered.

Brendon stated firmly, "Anything past kissing. Even kissing can be considered 'the road to sex.' If you think you don't need boundaries, then you're fooling yourself." He continued, "Unless you are relying on God's grace and accountability with others to sustain you, then you have set yourself up for failure. Someone told me that you can see temptation in the physical area as a pothole in the road, and I need to set up traffic cones around it. We need to be honest with ourselves to know what we are going to struggle with."

Garret admitted, "It's hard. Early on in dating guys tend to be more physical than girls. Don't let us! I think it is appropriate to talk about the boundaries, but I don't think it's easy. The way a girl dresses can help or hurt us. Don't do that! Watch the signals that you send, watch what you wear."

"How can girls help us?" asked Bradley. "We both must clearly set the standards and expectations *before* going into the relationship, not trying to 'play it by ear' or address the issues as they come up.... Make sure your motives aren't selfish. And set clear boundaries for yourself that you share with a third party (such as friend, pastor, or father) whom you trust to step in if those boundaries are crossed."

Robbie concurs:

It has to be a commitment by both parties. Sometimes girls feel like they need to give themselves sexually to keep guys, but that is the furthest thing from the truth. It is better to be mysterious than to reveal everything! If a guy is going to leave you because you don't have sex, then that's a guy you don't want! There are plenty of other ways to keep guys interested without doing that. People respect those who "hold the line."

The Bible says, "abstain from every form of evil" (1 Thessalonians 5:22, NASB). You don't want to put yourself in situations (like being alone in a dark house) in which you can be easily tempted to do bad things.

Jeff suggested the obvious: "Keeping your clothes on is always a good one. And being alone in a bedroom is dangerous. Nothing good can come out of that. It's too inviting. You can have a conversation ahead of time, explaining why it is bad from your perspective and from God's perspective. But boundaries can be easily forgotten in the heat of the moment." Then he shared, "In my

TOP TEN THINGS GUYS DO TO KEEP THEIR MINDS OFF SEX

(from a guy friend of mine who shall remain nameless)

1. Eat everything in the fridge.
2. Go for a long jog.
3. Walk the dog.
4. Go to a sports bar (*not* Hooters!) and eat hot wings.
5. Play video games.
6. Wash the car.
7. Mow the lawn.
8. Go hunting or play paintball.
9. Go skydiving.
10. Babysit someone else's kid.

experience, it has always been the girl who has crossed the boundary first. When I've called it out, she said, 'You really don't want to be with me,' and then it became an emotional thing."

So it takes a commitment on the part of both people in the relationship to really make a go of it. Shawn concludes, "We need to set physical boundaries, then communicate with one another and honor one another—and God—in that. When you follow through with the plan, you don't have to overanalyze everything. You can be free to just trust God and go with it, rather than live in fear that something bad will happen."

PHYSICALLY SPEAKING AND FACEBOOKING

I wanna know why some guys only look on the outside for beauty. Not everyone is a swimsuit model!

—*Vanessa*

Do guys like girls better with makeup? I don't wear any and guys still like me. So I wonder why girls obsess over it.

—*Charlene*

Why is it that appearance *always* wins out over character?

—*Sharon*

Men do look at the outside first most times. I heard comedian Steve Harvey saying that women engage in sex too soon (i.e., before marriage), they lower their expectations instead of keeping them high so that the right guy rises to meet them. He says, just like on a new job where you have a ninety-day probation period, you should give yourself the time to get to know the person.

—*Manuel*

Given a choice of two girls, both godly in their own ways, and one is slightly less attractive or not as thin as the other, which one would the guy be likely to pick as a mate?

—*Paula*

Do guys scout out other girls before deciding on one?

—*Elizabeth*

Why do looks matter more than personality traits? Isn't personality what matters most in a relationship/marriage? Why are guys so judgmental anyway?

—*Keri*

A man wants a woman who maintains physical attraction as well as spiritual attraction.

—*Chad*

What is an absolute deal maker or breaker, as far as whether or not you would pursue a relationship with a girl?

—*Bethany*

For me, a Christian lady is number one, and being a non-smoker is number two. She could look like a supermodel, but if she doesn't meet these two qualifications, I would not even consider her as a candidate for dating. Looks are somewhat important— there has to be an attraction—but there has to be something deeper.

—*James*

I echo the statement that a mature Christian guy will look for more than physical attraction. The Bible warns against that kind of thing a lot; "beauty and charm are fleeting, but a woman of noble character is to be praised!" If Christian guys don't get that, they're going to end up alone, or worse, stuck in something they're unhappy in.

—*Lindsey*

Why do guys claim they want a girl who dresses modestly, then date the one who is slutty?

—*Rachael*

Guys, one of my questions would be: What does God's holiness mean to you? How do you apply this in your daily life? A lot of a guy's behavior and attitude falls under this, especially what he does with his eyes.

—*Karla*

I know what guys are thinking—same things they always did. Wish they were more romantic and would take time to get to know a girl. If they get hurt it's 'cause fools rush in. It takes time to know someone. I will stay single from what I know about men.

—*Mandy*

I wish I had known what I know now about what most men are thinking—sex. I wish I had saved my virginity. I wish I had truly listened to God. I wish I had known about the dynamics of relationships and how it is so common for couples to think that the love of each other can heal brokenness and free baggage. I wish I had known that only God through Christ can restore us and make us whole.

—*Anonymous*

Do single Christian virgins still exist anymore in this depraved world? I am coming to believe they don't, because many "Christians" want sex before marriage. It's happening a lot at our church. I wish I could find a Christian guy who's really Christlike.

—Michelle

In what ways do we dress that can be a temptation to you? My friend's boyfriend says that certain things (that seem harmless to us girls) can turn a guy's mind the wrong way.

—Theresa

Can you give us more specifics on what we wear that causes you guys to sin? Because sometimes we just haven't got a clue!

—Melanie

I wish guys would consider setting a time frame for simply getting to know one another—no physical stuff—so there would be a fair chance of actually figuring out if you are compatible without getting confused by lust!

—Lily

STAYING PURE IN MIND

It's no secret that guys are visually stimulated. That's why temptation is such a huge challenge for them. I was curious if there was anything women could do to help them succeed in being godly in this area—so I asked.

Brendon answered, "Be sensitive that guys are visual and touch oriented. Realize that what you are wearing does affect how we think and our minds take things way farther than is reality. Discuss

---

THREE WAYS TO GUARD YOUR THOUGHT LIFE

1. *Take control (2 Corinthians 10:5).* You may not be able to control every thought that comes in, but you can determine whether or not it stays.
2. *Guard your gate.* What's the gate of your mind? It's your eyes and ears. Filter what comes in.
3. *Thought replacement.* When thoughts of fear or doubt come your way, replace them with love and faith. For good thought replacement ideas, see Philippians 4:8.[2]

---

the boundaries together. A guy should be able to say, 'This is what I can handle. This is what I *can't* handle.'"

Andrew explains, "Today, marketing is predominantly done in three ways: 1) a really good product just sells itself; 2) comedy is used; and 3) sex sells.

"Some girls are shocked at just how visual guys really are. Physical temptation is a massive struggle for all guys. Once women understand that they can help guys out by the way they dress and by what kinds of stuff (like Victoria's Secret catalogs and fashion magazines) they have around the house."

Proverbs 4:23 says, "Above all else, guard your heart, for it is the wellspring of life." The apostle Paul promises in Philippians 4:7 that the peace of God "will guard your hearts and your minds in Christ Jesus." Many guys do want to make conscious decisions to guard their hearts and minds from sexual temptation. Here are three ways that my friends have discovered to do that:

1. "I've made a personal commitment not to get on the Internet alone. It's not that I don't trust myself, but why knowingly put myself in a position where I know I'll be tempted?"

2. "I have an accountability partner whom I am completely honest with about my struggles and weaknesses."
3. "By keeping God at the center. I don't allow myself to get into vulnerable situations (late at night at a girl's house, for instance). I try to stay away from the line."

The goal for them is to please God by living with a clean conscience before Him, knowing that He is watching. And that's a goal for which women should be striving as well. It used to be that guys were the ones who mainly struggled with pornography. Now, in our massively oversexualized society, many girls are directly facing this temptation too. Consider, for instance, these facts:

- Nielsen NetRatings reports that nearly one-third of the visitors to adult websites are female.[3]
- One out of every six women, including Christians, struggles with an addiction to pornography. That's 17 percent of the population, which, according to a survey by research organization Zogby International, is the number of women who believe they can find sexual fulfillment on the Internet.[4]

I asked a couple of my guy friends, "What would you say to encourage girls to stay away from pornography?" Nathan said,

Due to the way the world has idolized porn stars, it is often hard to remind ourselves that pornography is a pit of destruction. There is no good in it. Any girl struggling with any form of pornography needs to question what she is truly longing for, and look at pornography as the distraction that is pulling her heart's desires away from that core longing. There is a hunger that is being squelched, and pornography tends to pollute our minds and add a heaviness to our hearts that is hard to shake off. Because people's struggles with pornography are widespread today, finding support is not hard to do. Just know, the deeper it pulls you in, the harder it is to engage what you are meant to receive from God. He longs to give freedom in this.

Brendon shared, "We were created for true and whole connection with God and with our mate. Pornography is a counterfeit for love and will leave participants scarred and empty. Porn is a dead-end street."

Julian agreed,

We're hardwired to experience intimacy with our Creator, and with each other, in the context of healthy community. Sexual intimacy was designed to be enjoyed between a husband and his wife; pornography is a counterfeit to true intimacy. If women are turning to a counterfeit, it's because they are not experiencing fulfillment the way God intended. Sex between a husband and a wife is a blessing, but is not a substitute for the intimacy God desires to share with each of us. If a woman is struggling with pornography, I believe the answer to her freedom is found in relationship with her heavenly Father. He wants to satisfy her with His love and goodness, providing the security that can only come from Him. Psalm 107:9 says, "For He has satisfied the thirsty soul, and the hungry soul He has filled with what is good" (NASB).

Andrew had this to say:

I have a feeling that there are different motivations driving why guys are drawn to pornography and why girls are. How to stay away from it? I'd suggest a couple of things. First, don't even play with it at all. It has to be fought before a time of temptation comes. I would recommend taking preventative steps to protect yourself and your family from it by using a solid filter system on the Internet—such as Safe Eyes or Net Nanny.

Second, you have to make a conscious decision to not get caught up in it. Not everyone is willing to do that. Once someone is caught in this particular sin, it takes radical steps to get out of it.

Third, ask yourself the question, "What does it look like to be a godly man or woman?" Then, the follow-up question is naturally, "What am I willing to do to become that godly man or woman?"

Finally, I would say that community life is crucial. This is not a battle to be won privately. I have never known someone who has struggled with this and overcome it who has not had a small group of people who closely helped him (or her) to fight through it. This is a battle to be won—both before and after—by the community.

In addition to the wonderful challenges the guys have just given to us, I think it's a good idea to stay public when we're on the computer. Don't sit in your room for hours alone with the Net. Work online in the living room or at a café. Accountability works.

IS MODEST HOTTEST?

I love what Jon had to say: "Modesty is attractive. A girl is like a flower, and if you treat her right, she will blossom. The gift of a woman's body is precious. Through her modesty she shows a lot about her character and what she values—and that she is secure in herself."

Nick commented, "It breaks my heart when I go to a youth group and I see all these girls wearing very short skirts. The media is a great influence on them. People are so afraid of being alone that they will do many things to get attention. A girl is God's princess and modesty is a characteristic of a godly woman."

Julian said, "The way a girl dresses says something about the way she feels about herself. If she dresses in a slutty way, it indicates that she is using those assets to grab the attention of a guy, and that she is probably not very secure in herself. Truly *hot* girls don't need to show too much. It is evident that they are beautiful."

Brendon responded, "Modest is hottest! If a girl flaunts her stuff all around so that every guy sees it, that's not cool. If a girl is comfortable in herself and she finds her identity in Christ, then she doesn't need to seek attention from others in a very negative way. Guys are very visual, so be aware. If it's questionable, don't do it . . . showing your stomach, cleavage, too much leg."

Garret affirmed, "Girls who respect themselves don't dress the way that girls do that *don't* respect themselves (showing too much cleavage, showing too much skin, wearing skirts that are way too short or dresses that are way too tight, and not leaving anything to the imagination). Girls should be well put together, but not look like they're falling apart!"

I love that line! I asked, "How can women present themselves in a more modest way, and how is that attractive to you?"

Brandon offered this insight: "A woman who respects herself demands respect from me. I'd rather give respect than lust. Lust is something we all (yes, even Christian guys) have to deal with on a daily basis, and if it's our intention to honor God (not just physically, but with our eyes too), then you can help us accomplish that goal by not tempting us with your body in the way you dress."

Bradley concludes, "God has created my future spouse's body for me, and mine for her—as gifts to be enjoyed under the protection of marriage. I wouldn't want my Christmas presents to be left under the tree unwrapped for the whole month leading up to Christmas Day. It would devalue the gifts and ruin the surprise and enjoyment of Christmas morning. So, keep 'em wrapped until the right time comes!"

HOW FAR IS TOO FAR?

One of the biggest lessons I drew from asking guys about this topic is that there is a balance that needs to be maintained between godly boundaries and healthy sexuality. Though some people have a true sense of conviction that they are to wait until their wedding day to kiss, generally when girls tell me they're going to do this, I cringe! Personally, I can't imagine going from zero to sixty all on the wedding night. I dated one guy who had gone too far with the physical part of his relationships prior to dating me, so he had a conviction that he wasn't to kiss until engagement. I respected him for that and we held to it. But overall I believe that there is a way of being God-honoring and still being romantically affectionate in a dating relationship. God's strength, wisdom, and guidance must be sought in the process. He will show us how!

Part of the challenge for Christian singles is to own sexuality as a gift from God, yet not act on it until He provides the context (marriage) and life partner for which it was intended. We can be women of intrigue and mystery, as we've stated earlier. But it leaves us to struggle with the question, "How far is too far?"

In the name of purity, chastity, and good morals, *singles have been desexualized*. They are often repressed beyond normal decency, and as a result they are in a "presexual" stage of development—what psychologists refer to as "latency." In other words, *out of a fear of sex, they have regressed to preadolescents, and they are feeling and acting like twelve-year-olds instead of adults who have gone through adolescence and figured all of that out*. Getting shut off from sexuality causes a shutdown of the dating process.

When there is such a negative emphasis on sexuality, people fear their sexuality and get so out of touch with it that the sexual dynamic disappears from expression in their personality. They no longer attract someone of the opposite sex because their God-given sexuality has been turned off. There is little "chemistry." They dress it away, they talk it away, they preach it away, and it goes away.[5]

Dr. Cloud goes on to say, "I do not advocate sexual acting out. I advocate sexual ownership as a part of who you are."[6]

As a single woman, how do you do that? Where's the line that you should draw? When it comes to physical expressions of sexuality with men, what can you do in good conscience before God—and what shouldn't you do? Part of the answer has to do with physical boundaries, which we've already unpacked in this chapter. I was curious how guys would answer that question. Hear them out.

Bradley answered it like this: "I don't want to start down a road that I'm not prepared to finish. Rather than focusing on the physical aspect of a relationship before marriage, I'd rather focus on seeing if this person is someone I want to spend the rest of my life with. I'm looking for a life partner, not a bed buddy."

Brandon responded, "How far is too far? Anything that puts you in a position where it becomes easy to compromise the boundaries you have set."

Well, what if you've gone *too far*? Many young people that I have met on the road have expressed their pain over having sex outside of marriage. Having spoken about purity since I was sixteen, when I talk about this issue I always include some words about forgiveness. God does not want us to live in the past, but in the present, walking into the future with freedom from sin and guilt. I asked a few guys, "What would you have to say to a girl who has sexual sin in her past and is struggling with guilt?" Here's Nathan's response:

The Bible is so clear in its message of offering forgiveness for any sin. "Repent, then, and turn to God, so that your sins may be wiped out, that times of refreshing may come from the Lord" (Acts 3:19–20). I have felt many times that guilt was coming to me from God so that I would feel bad enough about myself that I would never sin again. When Christ was on the cross, He knew what He was dying for—and it included [the sin of] premarital sex. It pains Him to see us put ourselves in compromising positions that go against His longing for us, but there is tremendous power in the redemption that comes from Him "refreshing" you.

There is no place for guilt in a relationship with a loving God. Conviction? Yes. Guilt? No. The best thing for her to do for herself is to sit still and let God move in that guilt to bring her back to a place of security, peace, and an identity of being loved and nurtured from the most powerful love on the planet. [If I were the guy in a relationship with her] I would hope I would see her with the same eyes God sees me with—as forgiven, and deeply loved.

Julian offered these words of comfort:

I would tell her that God has made a way for her to be free from that guilt and everything negative associated with it—that there is freedom in repentance. First John 1:9 says, "If we confess our sins, He is faithful and just and will forgive us our sins and purify us from all unrighteousness." A great passage for anyone with a grieved conscience is Hebrews 9:13–14, where it talks about how, in the old covenant, the blood of animals purified people in need of cleansing. How much more will the blood of Jesus (a perfect, sinless sacrifice) cleanse our consciences? God is in the business of healing and restoration—spirit, soul, and body.

Andrew advised, "I'd recommend talking to a professional... a Christian female counselor who deals with issues like this on a regular basis." He continued,

> I think the place to really start with this one is Jesus. In John 8 Jesus had a fascinating interaction with a group of guys out for justice and blood when they caught a woman in some serious sin. Jesus did not take her sin lightly, but He told the woman He did not condemn her, then called her to leave her life of sin. Jesus isn't out to see that people get "what's coming to them." Instead He constantly calls people to repentance. He takes on the burden of sin and defeats it. Those who are in Him are freed from that past life of sin and death and brought into a new life. For those who have repented and turned from their sin (which is often a lifelong process) and yet still struggle with guilt over their past, Romans 8:1 promises, "Therefore, there is now no condemnation for those who are in Christ Jesus."

Brendon offered a great perspective on this. He said,

> If we are feeling condemned because of past actions that have already been confessed, we are listening to the enemy's voice. He loves to cause us to look back instead of looking up to the cross. It's one thing if we hear a voice convicting us of something we're currently doing that doesn't please God. But if the voice is telling us we're condemned and beyond forgiveness, that is clearly not God.
>
> Being in a place where we are well aware of our desperation for Jesus is a healthy place to be. When we realize we are in great need of the Good Shepherd it pleases God. We must believe the voice of truth over the voice of our emotions, if they are telling

us we are not forgiven. Beating ourselves up after messing up is saying that Jesus' blood is not sufficient. We can't buy what he already paid for in full.

Through my years of touring I have met so many women who needed to hear this message of grace and forgiveness. Please hear me clearly: if you have made mistakes in this area of your life, know that God stands ready to purify and forgive you. I was so very encouraged by hearing these same words from my guy friends about sex. I hear a lot of girls asking, "Why aren't there any godly guys around who have strong values?" Here is proof that they still exist!

A FEW TAKEAWAYS FOR YOU AND ME

———◆◆◆———

- Give dignity to your body and honor God by keeping yourself from sexual sin.

- If you build your relationship on the physical aspect, you will lose spiritual and emotional depth.

- Set your standards and ideals ahead of time.

- Talk to your boyfriend about physical boundaries.

- Don't take your clothes off!

- Guard your heart.

- Stay away from pornography entirely.

- Receive God's forgiveness if you've made mistakes in the area of sexuality.

6

Getting Serious

WHAT ARE THEY THINKING...ABOUT MARRIAGE?

"Give honor to marriage, and remain faithful to one
another in marriage."

—Hebrews 13:4, NLT

Years ago I had a show in Lexington, Kentucky. It was a
mother/daughter SHE event that our team puts on, centered around a book I have by the same name. Very early that
morning while we were sleeping, the bus had been parked at the
side of the church where we would be playing that evening. It was
a Sunday, so the whole crew went to church together. The pastor
was talking about families and he spoke about 1 Samuel 1:11 and
childless Hannah asking God for "a boy." When God answered
her prayer and provided one, she dedicated him to the Lord as she
promised she would. I really enjoyed hearing this story again and
found that the service had some takeaway points for me.

First, I started praying (like Hannah) that God would give me a
grown-up boy...a man! And second, I felt challenged by God that
when He entrusted this boy-man to me, I was to dedicate him—
and us—fully to the Lord. This is easier said than done when we

(like Hannah) want something, or someone, so much. It is a challenging thing to keep our relationships surrendered to God when we truly desire to be married. In our fear of being alone, we sometimes cling. Others fear being hurt or fear marriage and largely stay away from committed relationships altogether. Let's dig into this topic a bit deeper.

WHAT ARE YOUR ODDS?

According to the National Survey of Family Growth:

- Over 70 percent of men and women ages 25–44 have been married (71 percent of men and 79 percent of women).
- The probability that men will marry by age 40 is 81 percent; for women, it is 86 percent.
- A larger percentage of women than men ages 35–44 have married by age 35.[1]

Do you like your odds of getting married or not? And what if you never find Mr. Right? A woman named Danielle recently posted this on my Facebook page: "I was single until I was thirty-nine, so I know this to be true. You know a man is looking for a serious relationship when he's searching for a companion, not a trophy. A woman is ready when she understands the perfect man for her is not already married. To get her dream guy she needs to be looking for a diamond in the rough."

Guys have that same fear of not finding the one for them. My friend Jeff said, "The only thing I fear about marriage is marrying the wrong person."

One of my friends, Jon, chose to go the courtship route. Here's how he explained the differences between courtship and dating: "Dating is a one-on-one experience with an attraction usually being the main motivation. Courting is more about getting to know the person, getting to know one another's family. It seems more of a respectful thing in my mind. Sometimes in courting we have a chaperone, largely for the accountability. It can involve double dating as well."

I asked him how he started courting his girlfriend. He answered, "I talked with her mom and dad first, and asked them if we could court. We had been in groups together in the church, and I have known her since she was seven. I never dated anyone else and was never sexually active. I've waited a while and now we're going to get married."

I appreciate how he has been above reproach. Since age sixteen, I've been in a guy's world in the music arena, in the studio, and so on, and have always been very careful about striving to live with integrity. I applaud Jon's consistency and discipline.

Some women have not found the right guy because they've made it too tough on themselves. They have a sense of entitlement, in the sense in which nothing (or no guy) is good enough. Author Lori Gottlieb points out that there seems to be "a heightened sense of entitlement among women that previous generations didn't have. Our mothers might have wished, but certainly didn't expect, that their husbands would constantly want to please them, be attracted to them, entertain them, enjoy sharing all their interests, and be the most charming person in the room.... Many women today seem to be looking for an idealized spiritual union instead of a realistic marital partnership."[2]

Guys realize they might not find "Mrs. Perfect" either, so they don't expect us to be that. But they would like to determine after several dates if the relationship has potential to go further. Several of them talked about the shallowness of some girls around them, and how this ended the relationship. What are they looking for? Cale said, "I don't think it's fair to 'play with a girl's heart.' If I see myself being attracted to someone but I can't imagine myself marrying her, then I probably shouldn't be with that person in a romantic sense. It needs to end."

Bradley explained, "The girl I'm looking for has a love for God that far outweighs her love for anything or anyone else (including me); she exemplifies patience, purity, purpose, passion, and a love for kids."

ROADBLOCKS

Dr. John Gray explains, "When we feel a chemistry with a partner on all four levels—physical, emotional, mental, and spiritual—then we are ready for intimacy....

- *Physical chemistry* creates desire and arousal.
- *Emotional chemistry* creates affection, caring, and trust.
- *Mental chemistry* creates interest and receptivity.
- *Spiritual chemistry* opens our hearts, creating love, appreciation, and respect."[3]

Do you ever have trouble letting things go? Sometimes in relationships I can just go round and round in my head, analyzing whether this or that is an issue until I feel like I'm going crazy! In these times God has been teaching me to learn how to think things through and then to forgive and move on in my mind. My brother Luke, who also had this same tendency in dating to get "in his head," said that he learned to process things, take a note in his mind, and then put it on the shelf, so to speak. Otherwise he would withdraw from the girl he was dating and it would hurt their relationship. He couldn't stay stuck worrying about things. Forgiveness and learning how to let go and move beyond the hurts that come up in a relationship are so important to going to deeper stages in our relationships.

Referring to the stage of engagement between a couple, Dr. Gray points out,

We have the greatest ability to learn and practice the two most important skills of staying married: the ability to apologize and the ability to forgive. By practicing these two skills before the more difficult challenges arise, couples are then ready to get married. These two skills are like the two wings of a bird. Without both wings the bird of love and peace cannot fly ...

These techniques of apology and forgiveness can be used at any time throughout the five stages, but definitely they should be practiced as a prerequisite for marriage.... It is vitally important to know how to find resolution and compromise. Without the practiced ability to make up, you may eventually break up.[4]

I asked a few of my friends, "What have been the biggest roadblocks that have prevented your relationships from going further?" Brendon said, "Sometimes I've learned more about myself in a relationship with a girl. Other times the personalities didn't match up as well as I thought they would."

Robbie answered, "It's either been a girl who has jumped too fast or it has been that she wasn't very interesting. A guy usually chooses a girl initially based on how she looks. But that fades pretty quickly. The first date never tells you anything. I need someone who is intriguing and interesting and I can talk to for a long time."

Nathan spoke of a potential roadblock to a marital relationship being all it is meant to be. He said it has to do with unrealistic expectations of marriage partners. He says,

There has been a perception that once you are married you can detach from who you are and lean on the other person for all your needs. But the other person will never, ever meet those needs

---

SOME REASONS I HAVE BROKEN UP WITH GUYS

- I didn't trust him.
- He didn't treat me very well.
- He wouldn't commit.
- We had some different values.
- We each wanted different things out of the relationship.
- I wasn't attracted to him.
- He was too pushy.
- He wasn't strong enough.
- He didn't honor purity.

(Side note: The breakups were not a result of just one of the things on this list, but a combination of them.)

---

perfectly. Codependency is a marriage killer. It says, "If I'm married to her, then all my problems will go away, my loneliness will go away, and all of my fears, anxieties, and issues will all disappear." Regardless of whether or not you're married, those are all issues that have to be dealt with on your own.

FEARS

I had a conversation with Garret regarding the fears that single people have when they contemplate the prospect of marriage. Here's how it played out:

REBECCA: Are you fearful about marriage?
GARRET: Marriage is a scary thing. I want a wife who has parents that are happily married because I want my kids to see grandparents who are happily married. Divorce to me

is scary. And it seems that even in the Christian community there are lots of marriages just barely hanging on by a thread. Marriage is tough—it has to do with people spending too much time connecting with others on the Internet, spending too much time being married to their jobs, pornography, etc.

REBECCA: Selfishness is at the core of it. How much better would our relationships be if we were constantly trying to outlove one another, constantly trying to outgive each other, and really seeking to *prefer* one another above ourselves? And if we did this in dating relationships, it would carry over into marriage.

GARRET: We are so wired, yet we get disconnected from our families! Finances and lack of communication are big issues in marriage too.

REBECCA: There should always be more to explore about one another. Years ago I listened to a tape by Bill Hybels on the keys to relationships—and one of the things he highlighted was a teachable spirit. People should always have a passion to learn and grow. If both partners are committed to growing, their marriage doesn't ever have to become stale.

As I asked about fears, I learned that it's about much more than just avoiding divorce. Cale said, "I have fears of not being good enough. I think I fear parenthood maybe more than I do my ability to be a good husband."

In Nathan's words, "The church has put a bit of a demanding outline on guys concerning what spiritual leaders should look like. Too many men enter into marriage and lose sight of who they are outside of a husband and a father—they have been called into sonship with God the Father...and that's incredible! We are to live in relationship with Him, rather than just try to submit to His law in a very robotic and stilted way."

I feel that if a man will be passionate in his relationship with his God, his fears will take care of themselves. It is the same for us as women.

CAN YOU FIND WHAT YOU'RE LOOKING FOR?

Here are some more questions and comments about love for a lifetime via Facebook and Twitter:

Does love at first sight exist?

—Pamela

Yes, love at first sight does exist. The day I met my fiancée I just knew she was the one for me!

—CJ

Why would you date and plan to marry one of your ex's best friends? Is it love? Is it illusion? How long would you have to date someone before you are really sure, both of you, that it is God's will? Did you pray for it?

—Maria

How many guys out there really care and are seeking a lifetime partner?

—Dana

Do men ever pray about finding the right girl?

—Hailey

Single guys do pray for the right girls. And some guys are
not shallow. God help me to find the right woman.

—John

I totally agree with you, John. Ladies, you will know the guy
God has placed in your life if you are just patient and pray for the
man God has intended for you. Genuinely pray for this guy that
will be your lifetime partner.

—Bruce

We should ask three questions: 1) What is God's will? 2) What
is God's will? and 3) What is God's will for me? It's often not
what our flesh wants, or our logic. His sheep know his voice. His
sheep should listen.

—Jeffrey

As a young Christian man, I am trying to find the woman
God created for me. I am doing that by praying and waiting
on God. The woman I am seeking should have good morals
and character, love and put God first in her life, have a sense of
humor and compassion for others . . . just to name a few.

—Anthony

Anthony hit it right on the nail. That is absolutely true. I've
watched three of my best friends do this. They are so happy in
their marriages. They prayed and waited on God. I'm not saying
they don't have disagreements, but it was all done by God.

—Sheila

I have been with Christ for nineteen years. I am looking for a
woman whom I can pray with and share my faith with.

—Joel

I believe in the power of prayer and know that if people really listen and heed God's signs they will find their soul mates.

—*Stephen*

These days it's very well possible that you will stay single for a long time and maybe your whole life. It's good to prepare yourself for that possibility, whether you're a guy or girl. It's not fair to blame one gender for it. It's just the way of life these days. You can pray and maybe it will be answered, maybe not.

—*Bernard*

Why would we expect His blessing when we don't ask Him for His blessing? God decides when you will find him. And if you will be single your whole life, God will have a reason for that. We don't live for being married. We live to honor God. That's number one, and we must be focused on that.

—*Di*

Men need to hear and *listen* to the ladies' heart cries. I am not single, I have been married for thirty-one years and still get excited when I get to go home after work and see my love. **blush**

—*Shawn*

My husband shares things with me that kinda clue me in (although sometimes I wonder who needs the clue?!). A few days ago, we noticed a young couple playing Frisbee. My hubby says that most guys are usually playing just to be with the girl! Given the option, playing Frisbee vs. soccer with a girl— SOCCER! Apparently, the guys playing together are aiming to capture girls' attention! Who knew?

—*Judy*

SELFISHNESS... AND OTHER MARRIAGE KILLERS

I asked, "What are the biggest marriage killers today?"

Selfishness covers a lot of it. Sometimes people pursue things that they think will make them happy (like pursuing someone else on the side), and they find out that is a lie and won't make them happy. Money causes all kinds of difficulties in marriage, but that is also a result of selfishness.

—Brendon

Many people today have a fear of commitment. And people are just really selfish and are not willing to sacrifice things for the other person. We are such a me-centered society. If you like the person, then you should be willing to sacrifice for them, and if you are not willing to do that, then you probably shouldn't get married or be in a relationship with them.

—Cale

Selfishness! I had someone tell me that as soon as he stops having *fun* in a relationship he ends it. Marriage (and the pursuit of marriage) has no room for selfishness; you must always put the other person first.

—Brandon

Selfishness, lack of communication, and unrealistic expectations. Not enough people realize that love is a daily choice—not just a warm, fuzzy feeling.

—Bradley

MARRIAGE OBSERVED

Finally, I asked my friends, "What have you learned from watching your parents' (and others') relationships, and what do you think you might do differently in marriage?"

Brendon observed, "I've seen my dad be faithful. He has the most integrity of anyone I know. He is always putting my mom first above himself, and I really admire him for that. He seriously knows my mom. He does things all the time to make her feel special and valued. Another lesson I've learned is how important it is to be willing to compromise, to speak gracefully even in disagreements."

Andrew shared, "Marriage takes a lot work, a lot of giving of yourself. The marriages I perceive that are good are ones in which both partners are constantly pursuing each other. They never come to a place where they know absolutely everything there is to know about the other person. When we stop pursuing, we make assumptions concerning how people will respond—and that's not good."

Nathan explained,

A man is meant to be a true spiritual leader of a home, connected to his wife as a husband, connected to his children as a father, and connected to his God as a son. I see so many women who are the spiritual leaders of the home and they connect with their children so much better than their husbands do, so they take over and they dominate—and the man detaches more and more. So, in dating, pay close attention to the person across the table and question, "Is this gonna be someone who really steps up and provides the maximum capacity of what I need emotionally, spiritually, and mentally? Or is this gonna be someone with whom I'm just coasting because I'm so desperate to be in a relationship?"

"What would *I* do differently than my parents?" Bradley asked. "Hopefully nothing. My parents have been an excellent example of what a godly marriage should look like."

I agree, Bradley. My mum and dad have been awesome examples as well. It's time we turn our attention to some married guys that I know. They have so much to tell us about what they learned in dating and then in marriage. Let's see what we can find out from them.

A FEW TAKEAWAYS FOR YOU AND ME

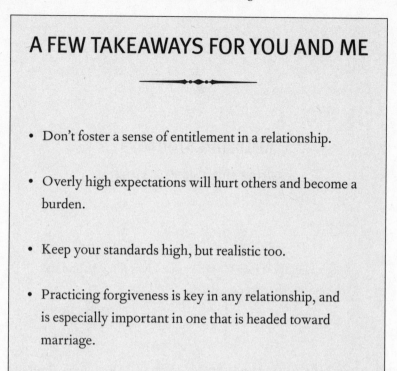

- Don't foster a sense of entitlement in a relationship.

- Overly high expectations will hurt others and become a burden.

- Keep your standards high, but realistic too.

- Practicing forgiveness is key in any relationship, and is especially important in one that is headed toward marriage.

- The number one relationship killer is selfishness.

7

Married Mentors
WHAT DID THEY LEARN?

"Each man must love his wife as he loves himself, and the
wife must respect her husband."

—Ephesians 5:33, NLT

Can I be very honest here? When I was first thinking
about this book and the content I felt it needed, I did not
want to interview married people about dating. My thoughts on
the subject went something like this: *They are married, therefore
they don't understand anymore what it's like being in the trenches of
dating life—even if they did only get married a month ago!* Hmm.
As passionate as I was initially about this, a few people spoke into
my life on the topic and it started to sound rather reasonable. Their
logic was that I needed to pursue some wisdom from those who
had actually crossed the finish line in dating because they would
probably have some good advice. Touché. Here's what I found.

FAMILY FIRST

My father David and mum Helen have been married for thirty-five years. I asked Dad, "What are the key elements in a great marriage?"

He answered, "Love unconditionally. That incorporates the small things as well as the large things. This means being willing to offer forgiveness on a daily basis. You need to be encouraging with your words as well as your actions. The core thing has to be deep friendship. With Helen and me, that has stood the test of time."

What do you feel you did right in your dating years with your wife?

I was relaxed in the friendship with Helen because I'd had previous relationships with girls that were more intense. At the time when I met my wife, she was very young, so the dating idea wasn't an option. It had an innocence about it, which looking back was very lovely. So with Helen it was more of a friendship than anything else. We built a friendship by just talking rather than going on dates. It didn't follow the traditional dating formula, so the growth of the friendship had a naturalness about it that I'd never experienced before.

What would you do differently if you were dating all over again?

At the beginning of the friendship, I probably wouldn't change anything, but toward the end of the dating relationship (before getting married), if I had my time again I would have made it less physical.

What marriage advice can you give?

It took me about ten years into marriage to start working it out. Looking back, I think I had too high expectations of Helen and too low for myself. I read a book titled *Inside Out* by Larry Crabb and that changed everything. The main challenge I got out of it was the importance of loving Helen unconditionally—which I started attempting to do. As soon as I did, I felt almost immediately that our marriage got better. It has gone from good to great. Helen wasn't too aware of my inner frustrations as she was busy with the kids—we had four kids in eight years leading up to our first ten years together.

I started to realize that it was no longer all about me. My goal daily—and I don't always get this right—is to put Helen first. I still don't have it all together but I try daily. Sometimes it is as simple as keeping my mouth shut when there is a potential issue. (I had an instance of that this morning when we got lost and were forty minutes late for an appointment.)

I caught up with my brother Luke and his wife Courtney right after they had returned from their honeymoon. It happened to be on Courtney's twenty-first birthday! They had some great advice on dating that you'll find in the next chapter.

You dated your wife successfully . . . what did you do right?
I have nothing but good memories. The thing I'm most proud of is that we had a good friendship before we started dating. The fact that we already knew each other and trusted each other made our dating life more enjoyable—and we were able to go through some heavy things together.

My uncle Ian, who is a pastor, has done quite a bit of premarital and marriage counseling. Here's some great insight from him.

What did you do right during your courtship days?
During our courtship I'm glad that we had a clear understanding of what is right in terms of physical intimacy. We both came to

our wedding night as virgins. I don't know anyone who has waited to experience sex with their marriage partner that regretted it, but I do know quite a few people who didn't wait—and regretted it. When my wife and I first got into bed with each other on our wedding night, it was a holy moment—God's blessing on our new life together. We highly recommend saving yourselves sexually for one another until you're married. There are a lot of regrets that can be avoided by exercising discipline.

What are the biggest relational issues you've seen in counseling?

The image of people being "unequally yoked" is an old-fashioned saying, but it is a very powerful image. It speaks of the impossibility of a believer having unity with one who doesn't believe. That is so important. If you marry someone who is not a follower of Jesus, it just doesn't work, because that is one part of your life that you can't share. Some things are nonnegotiable.

Another thing that comes to mind is domestic violence. When a girl is the center of a guy's universe, he lavishes gifts on her and wants to be with her and nobody else. Sometimes he begins to pull her away from her own family. She thinks it's wonderful—*he's obsessed with me*. But we might never be able to foresee what that relationship may fall to.

Things are not always what they seem. You need to be very careful, and check out people's backgrounds, and if there is any sense of bad-mouthing your parents or wanting to separate you from your family—you need to heed the caution signs. It must be part of the consideration and discussion.

What are the factors you see that have made marriages successful?

Be willing to not "let the sun go down when you are angry." When you're lying in bed back to back after an argument, someone needs to be willing to "reach out a toe" and touch the other person and say, "I don't want to be mad anymore. Let's get on with it." The thief comes to steal and kill and destroy (John 10:10), and we don't want to give the devil a foothold. Living out the fruit of the Spirit and doing little acts of kindness (even though they won't always be noticed) has a way of keeping your love fresh.

My cousin Matt Smallbone shared some advice in previous chapters, and he had lots of other great stuff to contribute here.

What do you feel you did right in your dating years?
I tried and tried to woo in vain. I eventually gave up and handed it over to God. Eventually Mary came to me with an admission of a crush. This really helped me trust God with our relationship. We never lived in the same town until we were married, so this kept things fresh and exciting.

What would you do differently if you could do it over again today?
I would keep a detailed journal of everything—how I felt, the things we did together.

What marriage advice would you share with the women reading this book?
So many people's lives become a train wreck within months of getting married. What goes wrong? What I do know is that you have to enter into marriage soberly. You will never understand the meaning of the word *solemn* until you take your wedding vows looking into the eyes of the one that you love. It is heavy stuff.

As each year passes, I am increasingly surrounded by friends in unhappy marriages. As a result, I have found myself deep in the trenches in the marriage-saving business. I've been blessed with a remarkable nine-year run of marital bliss. The failing marriages around me have caused me to consider what has gone so right for us...and so wrong for others. Without suggesting that I have even a clue as to why people struggle to love each other within the bounds of marriage, I think that I have figured out the two main things that Mary and I have done right.

1. We have made a lot of good decisions.

When we were first married, Mary was teaching and I was disappearing to minister around Australia for weeks at a time in an indie rock ministry band. She felt the pressure of being the main provider and was becoming miserable. So I wrote a resignation letter for her and gave it to her as a gift. I then stepped up to the plate and started providing for the family. (Tragedy averted.)

2. We have fun.

My dad begins every marriage counseling session with the question, "Are you fun to live with?"

I acknowledge that this is not the most sophisticated line of existential questioning; however, I suspect that it is the most important marital question of all. We are sensible with money and avoid stressing ourselves out. We never criticize each other in public or raise our voices. Ultimately though, fun and solid decision making gets us home. These two keys allow Mary to respect me, and her respect allows me to love her.

A man must feel respected and a woman must feel loved for a happy marriage to exist. And it's very important that God is the center of our relationship. Make the big decisions that need to be made, and start having fun with each other again. These two simple steps may well plot your course back to the harbor. You will need to be brave, but nothing of significance was ever won by the timid.

GOOD FRIENDS

Steve Conrad is a really good friend of mine. He used to play bass in my band and has been a member of a book club I was in for several years called the "Soul Check Society." He has taught me so much about the power of Christian community.

You dated and married your wife successfully . . . how did you do it?

I still am not sure how I successfully won the heart of my wife—I definitely got lucky! For us it was a long process, and the biggest thing that I did right (in hindsight) was to simply be patient and steady in my love for Emily. It was hard, because I wanted to move much faster, particularly in the early stages of our relationship. Emily and I were friends for many months before dating seriously, which gave her time to see my character, who I was. Once we started dating, it was a matter of demonstrating my love in big ways and small, showing her that I treasured and valued her. There were times in the early stages that I felt like I was further ahead and wanted her to feel as deeply as I did. But sometimes the heart of a woman takes longer to open and for love to develop. Many women have been hurt by guys who treated them poorly, and it can take time for trust to develop and for a woman to allow herself to love deeply. But when that happens, it is the most amazing and beautiful thing.

If you could do it all over again, what would you do differently?

I think I would try to be more "in the moment." When you're in a relationship that is significant or feels like it is heading toward marriage, it's so easy to think about the future. It's important to talk about the future, but dating is such a fun season—and one that goes by so quickly. Savor each moment of the process, and try not to let your mind race toward the future.

How did you keep your relationship growing deeper?

We were intentional about asking deep and important questions. We talked about books we were reading, sermons we heard, and things that we were thinking about. As we moved closer to marriage, we discussed what we wanted our life to look like together—the values that were most important to us, and how we would live out those values. We talked about things like family and adoption, mission trips to Africa, giving to church and other organizations, where we would live, how we would engage with our neighbors, and where we wanted to volunteer and serve.

What marriage advice do you have for women?

Before dating Emily, I never understood the importance of pursuing a woman's heart. I think that every woman wants to feel that she is valued and worth pursuing. In the early stages of marriage, it's easy to pursue because there are so many emotions and you can't wait to spend as much time as possible with the other. But over months and years, it's the little gestures that guys do day in and day out that speak deeply to a woman's heart and let her know that she is loved.

Ted Baehr is president of Movieguide. It is a powerful ministry that helps families find quality entertainment and much more. I have sung at the Movieguide Awards show and really believe that this ministry is helping encourage quality family films to be made in Hollywood. Even more important, Ted has a really great relationship with his wife!

What do you feel you did right in your dating years?

When I was living in New York, one year before I met Lili in Houston, God gave me a dream about her—whom I did not know and had never met. Then the dream recurred in San Francisco,

Los Angeles, and Sante Fe, New Mexico. It finally was fulfilled in Houston, Texas, when my movie production partner, Peter Graves, who became a VP of Warner Bros., met her briefly at the architectural firm where Lili worked. Peter told me that he had met the girl of my dream, because I had described her to so many people so very clearly.

I was dating the daughter of the owner of the architectural firm, so I called Lili to ask her if she wanted to go out with Peter. That night, when I met her it was as if we had known each other all our lives.

What would you do differently if you were dating all over again?

Nothing! It was all God's doing, and I praise Him for His grace.

How did your dating life mature?

Our relationship grew closer because of an extensive amount of prayer. After we were married, we went to Marriage Encounter, which was a great blessing. We both learned to strive to give a hundred percent to the relationship.

What marriage advice do you have for those listening?

My advice is simple: marriage is like two precious gems being thrown into a rock polisher. They are thrown up in the air by the circumstances, economics, and activities of everyday life—and they are polished by hitting against each other. The more precious they are, the longer they take to polish. If they are not precious, they grind to dust. They are finished being polished when God can see his face in them.

Don't give up. Be precious. Allow God to polish you.

Mark Hanlon is a vice president at Compassion International, an incredible child-sponsorship organization that I have had the privilege of partnering with through the years. Mark's wife recently battled a life-threatening disease, and I have witnessed these wonderful friends of mine draw nearer to God and each other in this time of pain.

Tell me about your dating years. What are some things that you did right?

We were friends before we were lovers. We were really good friends for about four years before we even started dating and subsequently fell in love. In fact, Joey knew all of my girlfriends— talk about full disclosure! As exciting and beautiful as the physical aspect of being in love is, you spend so much more time just enjoying each other's company in the big scheme of life. This really helps when you face hard times as a couple—and *you will face hard times*, whether it be relational, family, children, sexual, health, or financial. The Bible says that in this world we will have difficulties (John 16:33) and during these times, passion alone will not carry you through. It will be that unselfish, sacrificial, "fully committed to you" love for your best friend that sustains your relationship.

If you could do it all over again, would you change anything?

At times, as a teenage guy, I acted in an immature and selfish manner. I know I hurt some of the girls I dated by my behavior, selfishness, and attitude. I regret that and wish I would have understood then, as I do now, how my actions and attitude impacted them.

What marriage advice do you have to share?

My wife Joey and I just celebrated thirty-one years of marriage and we are so thankful for each one—especially after the last couple of years!

Quitting on marriage is not an option. You both must work to be fully engaged in the marriage and willing to invest in it and fight for it. This must be a basic value agreed upon by both the wife and the husband that they will hold on to during the hard times. There are exceptions, such as situations of physical abuse or lack of safety of children, but for most of our friends who have divorced, this is not even remotely the situation. They walked into the marriage thinking that getting out was an option and when they stopped loving one another, they quit. There have been times when Joey and I have found ourselves clinging only to our personal commitment to not quitting the marriage. It was the one thing that kept us fighting for the relationship.

Another thing, don't marry someone thinking you can change your spouse. I have seen too many young women settle for a guy they think can or will change after marriage. Rarely does that happen. In fact, more often than not, the woman takes on the negative aspects of the guy rather than the guy taking on the positive aspects of the woman. The influence and change often tends to go the wrong way. It's always easier to go downhill.

PASTORS AND MENTORS

Wess Stafford is president and CEO of Compassion International. I call him mentor, friend, and Uncle Wess!

Your wife fell for you and married you . . . how did you do it?

I'm not sure how much of this can really be attributed to what I did. It is probably more about how God prepared both of our hearts to meet each other. My trump card was probably that I fell very quickly in love with Donna and absolutely everything about her! She was very instrumental in bringing me to Compassion because she was a sponsor long before I had even heard of this place. Our first serious conversation was over a spaghetti dinner at her apartment while we were both grad students at Wheaton College.

I had just recently been hired to go work in Haiti, and Donna had agreed to tell me about her short-term missionary assignment there. On her refrigerator door was a picture of her sponsored child, and during that evening she described Compassion and all about Haiti, as well as her heart for the poor. Once I tasted her spaghetti, I knew it was a done deal! I fell in love with Donna, Haiti, and Compassion all in one evening—so clearly that it was a God thing. Right from the beginning, we knew each had a deep heart for God and the unique sense of the importance of the poor. In addition to that, we laughed together (I was a terrible tease!) and there was a real sense of just being comfortable, as if we had known each other far longer than we actually did.

What would you do differently if you were dating her again?

First of all I would choose a taller woman! Our first kiss was with me standing in the gutter and her on the curb so our lips could actually match, and that has been a problem in our marriage for the last thirty-one years. We rarely pass up a staircase! Before we had committed to each other and became engaged, I graduated and took off for Haiti, and we were separated for two years... I would certainly do that differently if I could. But distance does sometimes make the heart grow fonder. That was in the days before e-mail, so we actually wrote our deepest thoughts on paper (a novel idea!), and although our relationship was literally held together by postage stamps, it allowed us to get to know each other really well. In those days, telephone calls between Haiti and Chicago cost nine dollars a minute. I can remember conversations where we were both so choked up we would just sit and listen to each other cry for about three or four minutes at a time.

Eventually, my mind began calculating what this was costing me and I realized that a three-minute cry just cost me twenty-seven dollars and I couldn't afford to keep doing that. So I decided I had better just marry this girl! What amazes me is that, first of all, she would agree to marry me, but also that she would spend her life living among the very poor in Haiti. Ultimately, that was not God's plan for us, but I've never forgotten that she was willing to do that.

What words of wisdom do you have to share about marriage?

Like anything that really matters in life, it doesn't *just happen*. Marriage is first and foremost a firm, deep commitment, and then a lot of hard work. Put the option of failing completely out of your heart and vocabulary. "Until death do us part" means exactly that. You may go through deep valleys and rough patches and some of them might even last a long time; but if neither of you has "giving up" as an option tucked away in the back of your mind, the valleys soon end and the marriage will be stronger for having been tested.

Mark Foreman is the pastor of North Coast Calvary Chapel, in Carlsbad, California, the church I attended when I lived in San Diego a few years ago. His sons, Jon and Tim, are avid surfers and founding members of the band Switchfoot. Suffice it to say he's heard a lot of music in his house through the years.

Before your wife married you, what do you feel you did right in your dating years?

Jan and I dated for three years; still, I think we hurried things along. I wish we would have taken more time after graduating from college to just *be*, then get married. But we were in love and still are thirty-seven years later.

• I was authentic. Too often in dating people hide and put on their "best" to disguise who they really are. I tried to live with integrity so that what you saw was what you got.

• I exhibited a strong character of belief and action in regards to my faith. Jan says that my discipline was attractive to her. She understood that I needed time to pray and study. Sometimes we would do this together and sometimes apart.

• I was attentive to her by listening and genuinely wanting to know who she was.

• We did various things together so we could see all facets of each other: fun, study, prayer, groups, classes, families, and sports.

• I let her eat. All other girls I dated ate like birds and I had to finish their hamburgers. Jan ate it all. Picnics were huge. I knew I better let her enjoy what was rightfully hers. Seriously, we enjoy creating eating adventures, going and doing crazy things.

What would you do differently if you could relive your dating years?

I would have more playtime. Being in the thick of the revival of the Jesus Movement and going to college together created many serious conversations and moments. Then going into the ministry together at a young age kept us as serious little adults. Later in life we have had to learn to fight hard for play moments. We schedule dates now where no dumping of problems is allowed. We keep it light to develop the fun side of our relationship.

What marriage advice can you share with the women reading this book?

Dating is a gift of a period of time when you walk parallel with someone to investigate who he or she is in a fun way. To hurry the process is to stunt the relationship. Romantic love grows quickly, but that is only one aspect of a relationship. It takes time to discover attitudes and moods, intellect and imagination, dreams and hopes, character in all kinds of settings. It is the investment of a lifetime, and time must be treated as our friend, not our enemy.

We have an expression that states, "pay me now or pay me later." Either way you are going to have to pay. Find out who you are truly dating before the marriage. It's harder to find out after marriage. True love is saying yes to a person's faults as well as strengths. Dating often hides the faults, so time is necessary to allow them to bubble to the surface so that we say "I do" at the altar to *all* of who they are. Dating allows the fruit to ripen, and the fruit must not be picked too early.

Rick Anderson is an elder and worship minister at Mount Carmel Christian Church in Cincinnati, Ohio. I've known Rick, his beautiful wife, Barb, and their awesome kids for over fifteen years. They have a tremendous gift for leading others in worship—and it comes out of an obvious love for God and for one another.

During your dating years with your wife, what did you do right?
I can't take credit for it. After many years of trying to make "wrong relationships right," this time I let God handle it. I got to the point in my life where I felt more alone in a relationship I was *not* supposed to be in than I did when I was alone and had my relationship with Christ. I realized that He was the source of strength and contentment. When I finally ended a prior relationship, I prayed that God would introduce me to my wife or that I would be content being alone and having my relationship with Christ. Two weeks later, I met my future wife.

God did it, not me, and honestly, I believe that's how it should work. Any new relationship that has the potential to be as serious as marriage should be built upon a solid foundation forged by deep conversations. Make the effort to really get to know each other. Healthy boundaries should be established in order to help prevent physical interaction that tends to cloud decision making and leads to inappropriate relations.

What would you do differently if you could do it all over again?
I would try to wait on Christ and not be in such a hurry to date. In my opinion, dating and breaking up prepares you for marriage and

divorce. You should only date someone you would consider marrying. Courtship is the only thing that makes sense. I call it "dating with a purpose."

What marriage wisdom would you like to share?

I believe that in the marriage relationship the wife is "God's gift" to the husband and the husband is "God's gift" to the wife. If we keep that in mind, we will nurture, respect, and love our spouse in a way that is consistent with what Christ desires for us—and in tune with what He intends for marriage.

TALK, LOVE, AND SERVE

I had the opportunity to interview Sean Hannity, a very well-known TV talk show host, about marriage and family. I've had the opportunity to be on his show on Fox News quite a few times and he's a friend and "big brother." He said some profound things that I think are very applicable to our lives as believers—as single adults or as married partners.

Tell me about the dating process with your wife. How did it happen?

From the day my wife and I met to the day we were engaged was three months. From the day we met until the day we got married was six months. We've been married now for eighteen years. I led spiritually in the relationship. We did it the right way.

What marriage advice would you like to share with those who will read this?

I recommend that you look for little weaknesses while you're dating, because they will probably be compounded over time. Once you're in a marriage, overlook the faults of your spouse.

You should talk about everything that you think will come up in marriage *before* you are married. Do you believe in God? What church do you want to attend? What are your opinions about sex, about raising kids, about how many kids you want and how you want to raise them? Talk it out ahead of time so you both know what you are getting.

In marriage, I don't hide things from my wife. Everything is always out in the open. Be honest, make it fun, have a sense of humor, share values. That is *really* important.

Many people I see are looking to be served in their marriages, rather than looking to serve the other person. But true love is all about giving to another person.

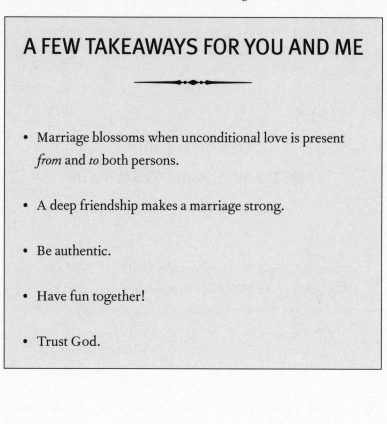

A FEW TAKEAWAYS FOR YOU AND ME

- Marriage blossoms when unconditional love is present *from* and *to* both persons.

- A deep friendship makes a marriage strong.

- Be authentic.

- Have fun together!

- Trust God.

8

An Open Floor

WHAT DO GUYS WANT TO SAY TO US?

"You will grow as you learn to know God better and better. We also pray that you will be strengthened with all his glorious power so you will have all the endurance and patience you need."

—Colossians 1:10–11, NLT

I hope that you've learned a lot about yourself and about what guys are thinking as you've come along this journey with me. It's amazing the life lessons that God sends our way if we are open to hearing them. Many of them come from the Bible, as we learn to apply His truths to our lives. Other lessons come from family members and friends around us who know us best and love us most. Sometimes life lessons come from a news story we've heard, a book that we are reading, an incredible journey we've taken, or a movie we've just watched. For instance, I stumbled upon a fun list, written by a guy named "Lobo," an ex-Marine who is married to a "wonderful wife," and has five "great kids." He presented this list of...

My 10 Favorite Movie Quotes: Life Lessons Learned Over Popcorn

1. *"What we have here is a . . . failure to communicate."*

This memorable quote from *Cool Hand Luke* was spoken by the captain of the prison work gang where Luke (played by Paul Newman) has been a constant thorn in his side. Many parents identify with this truism.

2. *"As you wish."*

This line from *The Princess Bride* was actually delivered by two actors, Cary Elwes, who played Westley, the poor farm boy in love with the lovely Buttercup, and Peter Falk, who played the grandfather. This phrase epitomizes what we feel when we deeply want to make those we love happy. It can be used to avoid arguments, provided it isn't spoken sarcastically.

3. *"I will take it! I will take the Ring to Mordor, though I do not know the way."*

Frodo Baggins said this in *Lord of the Rings: The Fellowship of the Ring*. As others argued about who should be charged with this huge task (which no one really wanted) Frodo spoke up, eventually shouting to be heard. He made a commitment to a task he was convinced would lead to his death, but he took it on anyway. We would do well to remember this when we're asked to do something when we're tired, have other plans, or just plain don't want to do it.

4. *"One thought he was invincible, the other thought he could fly . . . they were both wrong."*

Actor Steven Seagal spoke this as retired DEA agent John Hatcher in *Marked for Death*. Burned out from fighting a losing battle to stem the seemingly endless supply of illegal drugs, Hatcher retires—only to discover his hometown is being overrun by drugs and gangs. This statement deals with the futility of man's striving apart from God.

5. *"Honor is a man's gift to himself."*

In *Rob Roy*, Liam Neeson, as Robert Roy MacGregor, defines *honor* for his sons when they ask him what it is. If we believed this, and lived our lives accordingly, imagine how much better the world would be.

6. *"In order to find his equal, an Irishman is forced to talk to God."*

In the movie *Braveheart*, William Wallace had just asked Stephen, the Irish fighter, if he talked to God. Obviously we cannot claim equality with God, yet He came down to earth in the form of man to meet us where we are.

7. *"You put your hands on a child, all you get is dead."*

This line comes from Kris Kristofferson in the western *The Tracker*. A former lawman called out of retirement to track down a gunslinger, Kristofferson's character reminds the outlaw of the preciousness of children.

8. *"Dreams die hard and you hold them in your hand long after they have turned to dust."*

Spoken by Dennis Quaid in *Dragonheart*, this speaks to that sad, lonely part of the heart of anyone who has ever watched a dream die.

9. *"First learn stand, then learn fly. Nature rule, Daniel-san, not mine."*

Mr. Miyagi, played by Pat Morita, delivered this line in *Karate Kid*. In our fast-food culture we want everything and we want it now. This addresses our great need for learning both patience and perseverance.

10. *"It's not enough to marry goodness, you have to find it in yourself."*

In the movie *My Life*, actor Haing S. Ngor plays Mr. Ho, who works with Michael Keaton's character Bob Jones to help him deal with his anger toward his incurable cancer. This also speaks to the character of the person we marry, and what we can bring into the relationship ourselves.[1]

Life lessons can come from the strangest of places—from our own experiences and from stories of people we have never even met. I embarked on this journey with some preconceived notions, but also with some honest questions concerning what guys are really thinking when it comes to love, sex, dating, and marriage. Some of the things my friends shared about I quite expected. Others were a bit of a surprise. I heard lots of fun—and touching—stories along the way. I discovered some new things about myself. I hope that is true for you as well.

EXPECTATIONS

If you're a girl who is anything like I am, then you have probably at some stage in your life bought into this fairy tale: *When I meet "the one," we will fall easily and perfectly in love and then it will be marriage, babies, and happily ever after. It's gonna be just like the movies and the books . . . we might encounter a little trial or two on our way to wedded bliss but it won't be anything terribly challenging, just enough to make the payoff of the proposal even more romantic!*

I have asked dozens of married couples about their stories. Almost none of them sound like the fairy tale above. Some weren't really attracted to their spouse when they first met. Some broke up for a period of time before getting engaged. Some met online through a dating service. Every story is different and unique. There is no regimen to follow. No perfect way. In fact, I daresay that if you're looking for perfection in dating, you will never get married. This is primarily because none of us is perfect.

I am learning that the main ingredient in a great relationship of any sort is—are you ready for this?—grace. I need it, the guy I'm with needs it, and we both need it from God—so we can show it to each other.

I learned a big lesson along these lines through one of my dating relationships. Let's call my guy Jason. I felt that Jason and I were pretty perfect for each other. We brought out the "kid" in each other; enjoyed a lot of the same things; had very similar hearts for God, ministry, and family—and were very attracted to each other. It was pretty much perfect. But in my mind, our communication was not up to par. I thought we should be able to talk nonstop for hours on the phone and in person and never run out of things to say. *It should just flow*, I thought. *Our conversations should just about always be fun, witty, and deep. I should feel closer to him at the end of each conversation.* (Even as I write this, I realize how ridiculous I sound!) I hadn't consciously thought about these expectations beforehand, but my disappointment after quite a few of our chats—especially ones on the phone—was evidence of unmet expectations. A friend of mine calls it the "dreaded *E* word." Oh, the distress of living in the world of *should*.

- But shouldn't it be like this or that when you're in love?
- I think it should be more like so and so's relationship . . .
- I should try harder. He should try harder. If he really liked me he probably would.
- But shouldn't it just all come naturally?

I'm not so sure anymore. It seems to me that dating and the movement toward love takes a lot of honesty, a lot of grace, and a lot of prayer!

In her book, *Marry Him: The Case for Settling for Mr. Good Enough*, author Lori Gottlieb shares:

According to the most recent Census Bureau report, one-third of men and one-fourth of women between 30 and 34 have never been married. These numbers are four times higher than they were in 1970. At first, this might look like a positive trend—people are more mature at the age of marriage now. But many single women I talked to feel differently....

A barber in Montana said, "I have boatloads of eligible men as clients, but many of them have told me that they're ready to write off dating entirely. They say that the modern American woman brings nothing to the relationship except this deep-seated hunger for him to be her everything—unless something better comes along."

Or as a 29-year-old single dentist in Atlanta put it, "Women are always asking, 'Where are all the good guys?' And I say, 'You can't see them with your nose in the air.'"

Maybe we need to *get over ourselves*.

Barry Schwartz, professor at Swarthmore College, said, "You're continually looking over your shoulder to see if there's something better. And the more you look over your shoulder, the less good you'll end up feeling about your partner or a potential partner—even though he's probably just as good, on balance, as the people you're looking at."[2]

God taught me two big things through my relationship with Jason. First, my expectations (of him, of myself, and of us) were way too high. In a good relationship, certain aspects of your friendship (like communication) grow over time, especially as you learn to trust each other more.

The second thing that I needed to learn was to chill. To let go. To stop trying to control and *maximize* the relationship. Most guys are pretty in tune with the underlying pressure we put on ourselves, on them, and on the relationship. As I relaxed with Jason and let my expectations go (a form of grace), our conversations took an amazing turn for the better.

A NEW MODEL

Some women feel rejected because they've wondered why they haven't been "asked out," when in fact there has been a change in the dating ritual—and girls don't need to feel rejected. Some of my friends have asked, "Where have all the strong guys gone? Why don't men step up?"

One of the really big-picture lessons that was brought home to me through these interviews was that a new model of dating has emerged. Rather than guys just calling girls for dates, an organic and community-focused movement has come to the forefront. It is revolutionary and has happened over time. It happens in a natural setting and arises out of friendship. Garret called it "Starbucks dating vs. formal dating."

This relational model is much more relaxed. It helps take some pressure off. Without knowing that the model has shifted, girls have gotten angry about it, and that has put a chip on their shoulders and made them more distant—which in turn has continued to make building quality relationships difficult for them.

Nick points out, "A lot of people today simply play it by ear. With Facebook and all that, things are changing rapidly. There has been a shift to just let relationships happen organically. Don't rush into it, relax, and take your time."

Brendon observed, "Girls can dive into the depths of a relation-ship while a guy is still climbing the ladder to the diving board."

Did you hear that? Read that sentence again. We need to give guys time and space—or we'll simply chase them away.

Brendon continues, "Take it slower. Enjoy the fun of being liked at least for the first few months. We tend to be too calculat-ing. We need to just chill out and see what God does with it."

In Andrew's words, "We were made to be in a relationship with one another. Being on the same page, being in similar spots, and at the same stage of life is so important for success. Take time to develop the relationship; there should be a mutual pursuit and investment of time in one another. You should feel comfort-able being yourself in a good relationship. It's so important to be open."

I would add, "Get to know each other's friends and family by spending time with them. You learn so much about the other per-son within the context of a group setting. It's very insightful, see-ing how he treats and engages my friends and family."

Brendon comments, "It's important for each person to com-municate all along the way, like after a few dates. Something like, 'Hey, I'm interested in you, but I'm looking to take things slow.'"

Garret summarizes,

The way we approach dating is a lot different the older we get. Because of the high divorce rate and the way our culture depicts marriage, I think we are taking a more cautious approach. The dating is still intentional—but it's at a slower pace. All the more we want to really get to know the person first.

Part of that process is spending more time with groups. Because of social networking, we are all linked in and connected, and I think this plays into it as well. The "hanging out" period is much longer than it has ever been. This is where girls might get confused. Most guys are slower about getting serious because we are comfortable in this "friend zone." Being noncommittal and not feeling pressured is pretty standard for most guys. I think a lot of this stems from where marriages are today—which is not a good place. There is a safe haven here.

THE NEED FOR GRACE

For a long time, I was scared about hurting the guys I dated. But I've come to see that God can use hurt and pain to propel us into a deeper relationship with Him...not that I'm trying to be a catalyst for pain in a guy's life. But both people know that potential hurt is a risk one takes in a dating relationship. That's assumed. We can't let fear stop us from enjoying friendship and seeing what God wants to do in our interaction. It could be that we are just called to travel with each other for a season, and there can be much good in this. One of my relationships in the last few years was only three months long, but it was something that was very healing and empowering even though it didn't work out long term.

Vulnerability, openness, and deep sharing invite community. When we are vulnerable with one another, we see their humanity and we are drawn to them. Humanity links us together. We don't have to put on a big show. When I'm in a truly vulnerable situation and pouring out my heart, it can be so painful. It can hurt to be that vulnerable. Love is a risk and it will hurt, but it's worth it! What comes from the good kind of vulnerability is that the other person can choose to accept and receive you in grace (in your strengths and in your weaknesses). And you can do the same for him. There's such a beauty in this.

Grace is at the top of my list of how we can honor one another in relationships. Don't think the worst, trust the heart; don't jump to conclusions, choose grace.

Picture grace like this. When someone hurts you, it feels like that person owes you something. He (or she) has caused you pain, so now it feels that he should make up for it by doing something good. Perhaps that's why we like to hear the word *sorry* so much, because it feels like the one who's wronged us is now giving us something, a gift of repentance. But what if we, the hurt ones, decided to turn the tables and gave something to the one who hurt us? I call that a grace card. A "you owe me nothing" free pass. Think about the impact of this in dating! Oh how it would help us girls, who (if you're anything like me) can be oversensitive! It would help us not to sweat the small stuff. How wonderful it would be if we, because of the ultimate "grace card" that God has given us, offered free passes each day to one another.

Pickiness and a critical, fault-finding spirit turn us away from each other. But grace knits us together in trust.

SO WHAT *ARE* YOU LOOKING FOR?

My friend Andrew said, "In the past when I didn't know what I was looking for, it allowed me to become attached to some people that weren't the best for me. I wasn't actively setting up boundaries for myself. At times I was more passive and not as much the initiator as I should have been."

Lori Gottlieb explains that sometimes "what you want isn't necessarily good for you. And in going after the person you think you want, you ignore what you really need."[3] For instance:

You *want* someone creative.
You **need** someone you can trust.

You *want* someone who shares your love of jazz.
You **need** someone who appreciates some of your interests.
You *want* someone who is athletic and physically active.
You **need** someone who accepts you at your worst.[4]

I think the best way to take our relationships to a God-honoring level is to ask Him for his direction. Ask Him for his blessing. Ask Him to temper our expectations. Ask Him for his grace. Ask Him what we should be looking for.

My brother Luke and his new bride, Courtney, shared these awesome insights:

LUKE: If you only care about going on dates and having a boy-friend, then right from the get-go your relationship is going to be on difficult waters. But if you're looking for someone who can be there as a dear friend for life, you're not going to be interested in just having a boyfriend. It has everything to do with the way that you cherish and view your relationship. Approach it as though you are looking for a person with whom you can have a great chemistry, someone with whom you can pray and experience a deep relationship.

COURTNEY: Girls need to trust the guy they're with. Sometimes girls get stuck on what's next, rather than enjoying what *is*. You really just have to let go. With Luke it was easy. I really enjoyed him and just wanted to be around him. When you truly enjoy how God has made the other person, you can let go.

LUKE: When you are looking for the titles and the dates, it puts so much undue pressure on the relationship. Typically that comes from a place of insecurity. You might be looking to define something that may not actually be there at the present time. But you want it.

COURTNEY: I agree.

LUKE: While we were dating, we just wanted to enjoy each other and make memories together. Don't put unrealistic expectations on the other person. Don't make it any more complicated than it needs to be. Just approach it as wanting to be with that person, talk with that person, and experience new things with that person.

COURTNEY: You can't write your own story in your head. You can't control another person. Just let it unfold naturally. You don't know what God is going to do. After eight months of dating, Luke proposed to me, and it was a complete shock. I didn't write what he was going to do.

LUKE: When you allow God to lead your relationship, there is such freedom. It breaks down all sorts of walls and expectations.

PARTING SHOTS

In concluding each interview, I told the guys they had an open floor to talk with girls as if we were their little sisters. I asked them to share whatever was on their heart. Stein's advice was short and sweet: "Make a guy earn you, because that is how it should be. Maintain your self-control."

Here's some of the great stuff the guys wanted me to pass along:

Don't try to act like someone else to get someone to like you, don't be afraid to be yourself, don't share too much right away, don't be needy, don't be disrespectful, don't settle for second best (every good and perfect gift comes from God!). Don't text and call guys all the time. Don't be the pursuer.

Do give respect, talk, have fun, and set standards ahead of time. Become friends first. If you like them for who they are, let the relationship progress naturally.

—Jon

Nathan said, "No man will ever love you like God. There is no amount of human love that can touch what God longs for you to experience through His relationship with you. But man, when you get to a good place, it's a bonus to have an intimate relationship with someone you love."

Justin affirmed, "It all goes back to being faithful to God. Don't be stupid and make bad decisions because you're not in control because of alcohol or whatever. Don't date someone just to date someone. Don't be alone with a guy in his house and set yourself up for failure. Respect yourself and the person you are in a relationship with."

Twilight and *The Notebook* are not reality, and your life is not a movie.... Guys will say anything to woo a girl into letting them do what they want. Girls need words to be loved, and too many guys use their words to sweet-talk girls and manipulate and take advantage of them. So be careful! Unfortunately, a lot of guys have one thing in mind, which is sex. I would encourage girls to stay guarded. You can tell by guys' character, not just by their words, who they really are. Over time a guy will show you what he is made of.

—Brendon

Cale cautioned, "Be patient, don't rush into things. What you really want can wait. Focus on growing closer to the Lord in your faith. As your trust in God grows, He will provide you with what you desire and need. Seek first the kingdom and the rest will be given to you. Why would you want anything less than that?"

Robbie advised, "In the heat of romance you can fall in love with someone who is not right for you. Don't settle for things that are less than the best; make sure that the people you date get along with your family (or people you know who are looking out for your best interests)...bounce the relationship off them, and see what they think...then trust God and pray about it."

Be yourself and don't think this is your last hope of love. Relax and have fun. Learn to be friends. That needs to be there if it is going to go further. Enjoy each other's company and don't put too many expectations on the relationship. Be open and honest about what you are feeling. Don't have secrets, but don't be overly open either and let all the cats out of the bag.

Don't live in fear, and don't buy into the pressure that you have to do what everyone else is doing. Enjoy the time you have now and live in the moment.

—Julian

Pray to find a mentor who is a little older than you, who can advise you and provide some accountability. Do not compromise your desire to be faithful to God. When you honor Him with what you have, He will honor you. Don't rush. Relax. You want to be able to look your children in the eyes and say, "I waited for your dad." Do not give away something that is holy and sacred. Strive and hunger for righteousness. Die to yourself every day. Do not let the chains of shame and guilt haunt you and hold you back. Do not let someone else (besides God) tell you what you are worth.

—Nick

Garret encourages us, "Have fun with dating. Don't take it so seriously. Let it happen over time. Trust God, enjoy the journey, and see where it leads. Keep it interesting. Ask good questions. Find things to keep the relationship fresh, so that even if the relationship doesn't last, you'll have good memories. . . . And leave the baggage behind."

Andrew shares, "Protect your heart. I see a lot of girls who are so desperate to find a relationship that they compromise in all sorts of ways—emotionally, physically, and spiritually. Stand firm on virtue and stand up for what you believe."

> Don't settle. Listen to the truth of what the Lord speaks to you. Read His Word. Hear His words of truth that you are His daughter, that you are a precious gem, that you are a holy nation and a chosen people—and are deeply loved by the Creator of the heavens and the earth. He loves you. As you find your identity in Jesus, there is strength to honor Him in your relationships—to walk as Jesus walked and do as Jesus says. The more that you delight yourself in the Lord, the more the desires of your heart will be in line with the desires that God has for you (Psalm 37:4).
>
> —*Willie*

THE MARRIED GUYS SPEAK AGAIN

I asked my married friends the exact same question: "What advice would you give your daughter about dating?" Here's what Sean Hannity had to say:

> I don't see a lot of people out there who have conservative values like mine. Regardless of the kind of pressure that kids face today, the expectation is that my daughter should not have sex before she is married. She needs to know that the world does not share the same values as her parents. I want her to value herself—her soul, her mind, and her body as a temple and something sacred.

I don't see any relationship making it without some kind of foundation of belief in God. You need to have that anchor, that rock to stand on. Make a commitment to your principles and stick to them. You will face tough times, you will face tough challenges, you will have success, you will have failure, you will have joy, you will have disappointment. Nobody escapes the challenges and trials of life. And that's where shared values and faith will be what pulls you through and makes you part of the successful 50 percent that make it in marriage today.

I'll let the rest of the guys speak straight to you.

Ted Baehr shared, "Women and men should be guided in dating by seeking God's will. That does not mean to become hyperspiritual. It does mean to be sensitive to God's grace. The most important quality that the other person can have is that you enjoy being with them. This is a rare God-given gift. It is not about physical attraction, fame, or fortune. Love is deeper and more profound than all of that."

Be open to the idea that your love story may look very different than what you have pictured in your mind. Many of us (both guys and girls) have a picture in our heads of what our "ideal" looks like. We often write off people that don't look like the image we have created.

As my wife Emily often tells me, I was nothing like the man she envisioned herself with. But if she had simply written me off, we both would have missed out on an incredible love story. I am so thankful that Emily took a chance on a guy that was not what she had imagined. I think that she would agree that our story is richer and more beautiful than either of us thought it could be.

—*Steve Conrad*

Guard your heart, do not give it away too quickly. God has someone out there for you who will love and respect you the way you deserve. Pray for God's discernment and will for you. Focus on your relationship with the Lord. If you are not healthy in your relationship with God, do not be surprised if you are not healthy in other relationships. Someone who has not dealt with the brokenness within herself will have more difficulty being a positive influence on those around her.

Allow God to transform you from the inside out. Then watch and see what he does in other relationships in your life. Spend time with God. He loves you more than you can possibly imagine. Only God can fill the void inside of you. No man can fill your emptiness. Be whole and complete in Christ, then you can approach other relationships from a healthy perspective without putting unnecessary expectations on the other person.

—*Rick Anderson*

In addition to being friends (first), I'd say don't start dating seriously until you are at a place in your life when you are ready to get married. Getting into a serious emotional and physical relationship as a teen often leads to very difficult situations, decisions, and regret. So many things are still being formed in a person in the late teen years; it is hard to expect mature and caring behavior at such a critical time.

Use this time to find out what it is about a guy you like and dislike. But don't be too quick to give your heart away. Be vigilant about guarding your heart, because it is the wellspring of life. In the guys you do decide to date, find those who are honorable, courageous, principled, and who love the Lord—guys that you would be proud to be seen with beyond their physical appearance. If you see glimpses of those admirable qualities in them as young men, there is a better chance that they will develop those qualities even further as they become more mature men and husbands.

—Mark Hanlon

I have two daughters, so I have given this advice many times over the years. A guy will never treat you better than he does when he is dating you! If he does not open the car door for you when you are dating, he never will. If his humor is hurtful beyond innocent teasing and you feel "put down," you can expect a lifetime of that. Do not think that with your great wisdom and charm you will significantly change him. When you are dating, you are looking to uncover his heart, basic character, and godliness upon which you can build . . . *not rebuild*.

My daughters have often said when we've been discussing future spouses, "Daddy, we're looking for someone like you." And while that is very flattering, I have reminded them that this man that they see is not what their mother started out with. I am the product of what can happen when a wonderful, godly woman pours her love into the man God leads her to, even though at the beginning he is just raw material. Don't look for the finished product . . . look for the heart that can become "Mr. Right" with your touch.

—Wess Stafford

Be who God has made you to be. Because culture has placed the woman in a role of waiting to be asked out, waiting to be asked to get married, girls often suppress who they really are to complement the man. Although cultural things like that won't change soon, girls need to shine and be who God has made them to be. Shine in terms of personality, interests, activities, friends—and especially your faith. Don't hold back in hopes of "snatching" him. When the Bible says that "the two shall become one," it doesn't mean that the man is to eclipse the woman like the moon eclipses the sun. We don't become one by leaving who we are behind—that creates only a half. We must bloom and become who God has made us to be. Nothing is more attractive, and it allows the guy to know who he will be marrying.

Girls are first subjects of the King, and only secondly women who will date and marry. Develop your ministry and calling apart from whomever God brings into your life. Develop your career, friends, and interests. Become a healthy, well-rounded person apart from a man. If marriage comes your way, you will bring more to the relationship, and if it waits, you will live a vibrant life serving the Lord. Either way, He is glorified.

—*Mark Foreman*

My dad shared these final words of wisdom: "Check the guy's character and make sure that he's not a guy who's gonna take advantage of you. Talk to people who know him. Don't just date a guy you meet on the street—you have to *know* him. Start out with a friendship before you begin the dating process. Take it slow. Enjoy the friendship. Don't overanalyze. And be yourself."

Adventures are fun! I love to rollerblade, ride bikes, swim, camp, explore, see new things, go new places. In the heart of all of us, I believe that there's a longing for adventure. It's not just guys that love to live a new story and go on a journey. That's what dating can be, girls, an exciting adventure! And we have our Father God to protect us, lead us, and help us on our relational journey. Yes, it is scary at times and tough to navigate—but it is worth it! And God is shaping us in the process.

I hope you have been encouraged by my guy friends. I sure

have. I think after this, they're wanting to find out what *we're* thinking now! Keep being your mysterious, captivating, joyous, God-loving, peaceful, radiant, gracious, kind, beautiful selves— and let's watch God write the story of romance that He wants for you. Pray for God to "bring you a boy" and watch what He does. He will, for sure, take you on an adventure!

✦ Appendix ✦

SURVEY QUESTIONS

In case you get a chance to interview some of your guy friends, I thought I'd include the questions I asked my buddies and wise mentors. Have fun learning!

1. First Impressions: What Are Guys *Really* Looking For?
   - What are some of the most fun dates you've ever had?
   - Apart from physical attraction, what makes you notice a girl that makes her stand out?
   - What are the qualities you're looking for in a girl you want to date and might eventually marry?
   - How can a girl make you feel at ease on a first date?
   - What are some fatal mistakes girls make on first dates?
   - Have you had any embarrassing moments on first dates?

2. Understanding Guys: What Are They Thinking... About Us?
   - What are some things you wish all girls knew about dating and guys?
   - How does a woman you're dating make you happy?
   - What makes you feel respected?
   - What keeps you intrigued in a relationship?
   - What do you find annoying?
   - Can you give me some short "do's and don'ts" when interacting with guys?

3. Understanding Us: Flirting, Body Image, and Major Turnoffs

- What are some things you wish you understood more about how girls think?
- What don't you get about a girl's approach to dating?
- What have been the biggest turnoffs with girls?
- Have you ever felt pressured in a relationship? What did you take away from that?

4. Spiritually Connecting: God and Guys

- What do you think it means to honor God in a dating relationship?
- What are some good ways you've discovered that help keep a spiritual focus in a relationship with a girl?
- How can we each be dependent on God, not each other, for our identity?
- What does a healthy relationship look like to you?

5. Physically Connecting: Modesty, Sexuality, and Boundaries

- Why do you think so many Christians are trying to find loopholes in the command to stay sexually pure until marriage?
- How can girls help you with setting and keeping physical boundaries?
- What things do you do to work at staying pure in mind?
- How can girls present themselves in a more modest way, and how is that attractive to you?
- In your book, how far is too far?

6. Getting Serious: What Are They Thinking...About Marriage?

- What have been the biggest roadblocks that have prevented your relationships from going further?
- Are you fearful about marriage? If so, how do you deal with your fears?
- What are the biggest marriage killers today?
- What have you learned from watching the relationships of your parents (and others), and what do you think you might do differently in marriage?

7. Married Mentors: What Did They Learn?

If you interview married guys, ask them these questions:

- You dated and married your wife successfully. What do you feel you did right?
- What would you do differently if you were dating all over again?
- What marriage advice can you give?
- You have an open floor...what else would you like to say to us girls?

❧ Notes ❧

Chapter One: First Impressions

1. http://www.rr.com/dating/dating/article/rr/9392131/
   9392132/10_First_Date_Questions_You_Have_to_Ask
   (accessed August 1, 2010).
2. John Gray, PhD, *Mars and Venus on a Date: A Guide for Navigating the 5 Stages of Dating to Create a Loving and Lasting Relationship* (New York: HarperCollins, 1997), 15.
3. Dr. Henry Cloud, *How to Get a Date Worth Keeping: Be Dating in Six Months or Your Money Back* (Grand Rapids: Zondervan, 2005), 61.

Chapter Two: Understanding Guys

1. http://us.mc624.mail.yahoo.com/mc/welcome?.gx=1&
   .tm=1288539877&.rand=8rifbeoli6teu#_pg=showMessage&
   sMid=23&&filterBy=&.rand=1107635127&midIndex=23&mi
   d=1_18936_AFNLkoUAAVp6TFkXNA8snjRlzzk&
   fromId=funnies-owner@lists.MikeysFunnies.com (accessed
   August 4, 2010).
2. John Gray, PhD, *Mars and Venus on a Date: A Guide for Navigating the 5 Stages of Dating to Create a Loving and Lasting Relationship* (New York: HarperCollins, 1997), 133.

Chapter Three: Understanding Us

1. John Gray, PhD, *Mars and Venus on a Date: A Guide for Navigating the 5 Stages of Dating to Create a Loving and Lasting Relationship* (New York: HarperCollins, 1997), 317.
2. Ibid., 82.
3. http://www.nytimes.com/2007/01/16/us/16census.html?scp=1&sq=number%20of%20single%20women%20in%20America&st=cse (accessed August 6, 2010).
4. Lori Gottlieb, *Marry Him: The Case for Settling for Mr. Good Enough* (New York: Dutton, 2010), 31.

Chapter Four: Spiritually Connecting

1. Blaine Bartel, *Every Teenager's Little Black Book on Sex and Dating* (Tulsa: Harrison House, 2002), 3.
2. Arron Chambers, *Remember Who You Are: Unleashing the Power of an Identity-Driven Life* (Cincinnati: Standard Publishing, 2007), 11–12.

Chapter Five: Physically Connecting

1. Rebecca St. James, *Pure: A 90-Day Devotional for the Mind, the Body, and the Spirit* (New York: FaithWords, 2008), 106.
2. Blaine Bartel, *Every Teenager's Little Black Book on Sex and Dating* (Tulsa: Harrison House, 2002), 22.
3. Kathy Gallagher, "XXX Women Not Just a Man's World After All," *Create in Me a Pure Heart Blog*, 2007, www.purelifeministries.org (accessed October 31, 2010).
4. Ramona Richards, "Dirty Little Secret," *Today's Christian Woman* magazine. September/October 2003.

5. Dr. Henry Cloud, *How to Get a Date Worth Keeping: Be Dating in Six Months or Your Money Back* (Grand Rapids: Zondervan, 2005), 197.
6. Ibid., 198.

Chapter Six: Getting Serious

1. http://cdc.gov/nchs/data/databriefs/db19.htm (accessed August 7, 2010).
2. Lori Gottlieb, *Marry Him: The Case for Settling for Mr. Good Enough* (New York: Dutton, 2010), 131.
3. John Gray, PhD, *Mars and Venus on a Date: A Guide for Navigating the 5 Stages of Dating to Create a Loving and Lasting Relationship* (New York: HarperCollins, 1997), 91.
4. Ibid., 113, 126.

Chapter Eight: An Open Floor

1. http://www.associatedcontent.com/article/646737/my_10_favorite_movie_quoteslife_lessons_pg5.html?cat=40 (accessed August 8, 2010).
2. Lori Gottlieb, *Marry Him: The Case for Settling for Mr. Good Enough* (New York: Dutton, 2010), 45, 142, 150.
3. Ibid., 220.
4. Ibid., 221.